I'M MY FAVORITE

A Guided Journal for Your Path Forward

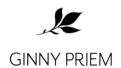

GINNY PRIEM

I'm My Favorite
Copyright © 2023 Ginny Priem
All rights reserved.

Library of Congress Control Number: 2023917798

ISBN: 979-8-218-23041-8

For more information from the author, visit www.GinnyPriem.com.

Book design and illustrations by Stefanie Geyer.
www.StefanieGeyerIllustration.com.

First edition 2023

I'M MY FAVORITE

A Guided Journal for Your Path Forward

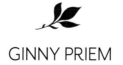

GINNY PRIEM

This book is dedicated to my unwavering supporters who have been and continue to walk alongside me on my own path. A special dedication to TB for being instrumental in the ideation of GINpath and DD for being the force behind bringing it to life.

I'M MY FAVORITE

A Guided Journal for Your Path Forward

GINNY PRIEM

INTRODUCTION

IN MY #1 bestselling book, *You're My Favorite*, I shared my true story of a traumatic and shocking experience of love, loss and learning that catapulted my healing journey and post-traumatic growth. It was in the midst of this process that I created and implemented the actions which I used not only to get through my experience but also to grow through, transform myself and walk the path to come out better and healthier on the other side of it: GINpath.

I'm sharing this process to provide you the same opportunity to transform your life, without the task of figuring out how to navigate this on your own. This guided journal is designed to provide you with prompts to begin to peel back the layers in order to better understand yourself and the adversity you have faced or are facing. It may also help you be more compassionate toward yourself as you begin or continue your growing and evolving journey. Finally, it can help you walk down the path of self-discovery & self-love and work toward building the life you deserve.

I'm My Favorite is the follow-up to *You're My Favorite* and is symbolic of your own journey. As you embark on your own path, you will be provided tools that can assist you in becoming the best version of yourself and your own first priority. This isn't selfish, I like to say it's self-ful. It's an investment in yourself, and when you're the best version of yourself, you show up differently. As the most authentic version of you, this is seen & felt by your entire community.

I'm My Favorite is an easy-to-follow guided journal. Use GINpath to rediscover who you're meant to be and the self-love that will propel you forward. Perhaps this journey will even help you discover these things for the very first time.

GINpath isn't a one-size-fits-all, prescriptive method. Rather, it offers options and suggestions within categories to customize your approach to growing through adversity.

You've taken the most important first step; you're here. Making a commitment to face your trauma, adversity or difficult times head-on to truly process and propel your life forward—instead of just getting through it or leaving it behind—is a huge first step on your path forward. CONGRATULATIONS!

XO,
Ginny

"YOU MAY ENCOUNTER MANY DEFEATS,

BUT YOU MUST NOT BE DEFEATED.

IN FACT, IT MAY BE NECESSARY TO ENCOUNTER THE DEFEATS

SO YOU CAN KNOW WHO YOU ARE, WHAT YOU CAN RISE FROM

HOW YOU CAN STILL COME OUT OF IT." –MAYA ANGELOU

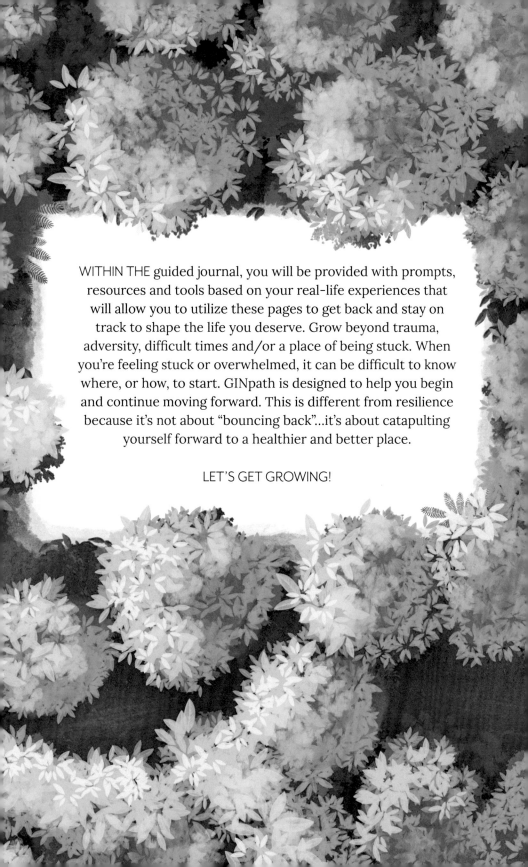

WITHIN THE guided journal, you will be provided with prompts, resources and tools based on your real-life experiences that will allow you to utilize these pages to get back and stay on track to shape the life you deserve. Grow beyond trauma, adversity, difficult times and/or a place of being stuck. When you're feeling stuck or overwhelmed, it can be difficult to know where, or how, to start. GINpath is designed to help you begin and continue moving forward. This is different from resilience because it's not about "bouncing back"...it's about catapulting yourself forward to a healthier and better place.

LET'S GET GROWING!

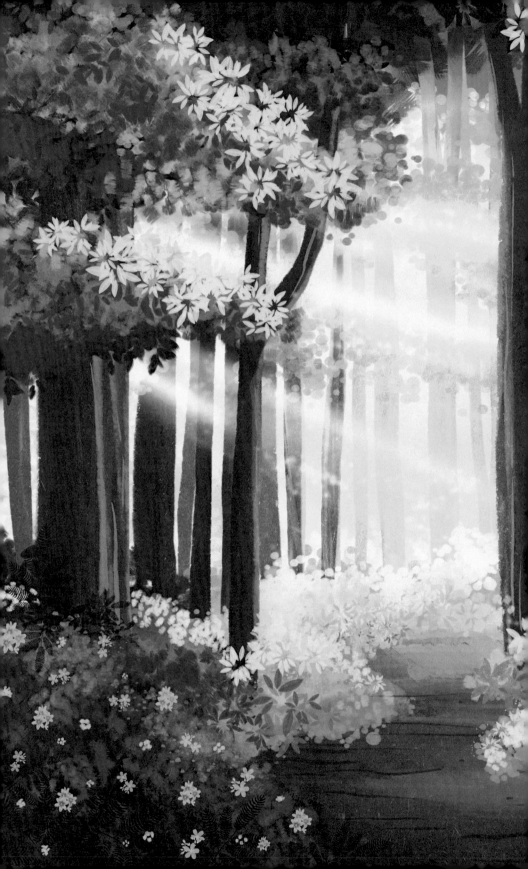

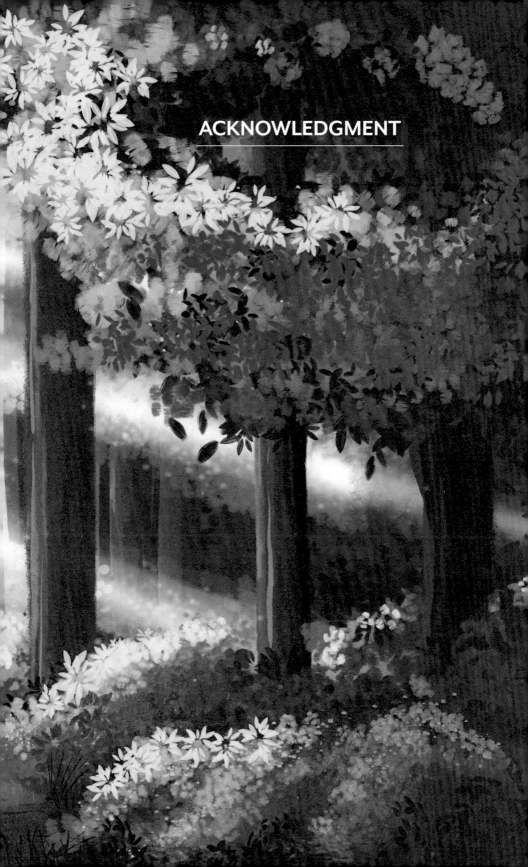

ACKNOWLEDGMENT

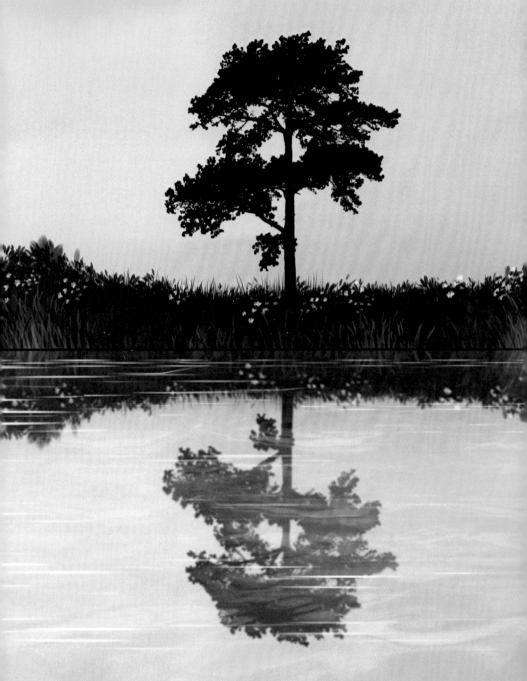

"You can't heal what you
don't acknowledge."
— Jack Canfield

DIFFICULT TIMES are inevitable. We all face them and have a story. You may not think your story is worthy of sharing or managing through. You may even feel embarrassed or silently carry around shame, guilt or stigma about what you went through—or might still be going through. Acknowledgment is an important part of the process because it prepares you for the path: GINpath.

Telling your story doesn't need to be out loud. I'm not suggesting you need to share your story publicly or with strangers. But I do recommend acknowledging it. Even if it's only to yourself here in the pages of this journal. Acknowledge what happened, where it took you and the path it sent you on. Recognize this as part of working through your experience and your path forward.

It's not always about what happened, but about what happens next. It's about overcoming adversity, trauma and difficulties to grow forward. And it begins with acknowledgment.

The journal prompts on the following pages are designed to help you acknowledge your story or situation.

WHAT IS the situation or circumstances that put you in the face of adversity, a traumatic time or difficult experience? This may include —but is not limited to— physical injury, illness, loss, financial issues, mental strain or emotional harm. What's your story?

USE THIS space to capture additional details about where you were, what you were doing and how this impacted your life. What other contributing factors or people were involved?

_____
_____
_____
_____
_____
_____
_____
_____
_____
_____
_____
_____
_____
_____
_____
_____
_____
_____
_____
_____
_____
_____
_____
_____
_____
_____
_____
_____
_____
_____
_____
_____

WHAT WAS your mindset at the time? Use this area to jot down the feelings you processed. Did you feel fear, anger, frustration, overwhelm, devastation, disbelief or optimism? What feelings are coming up for you now about your story?

_____

_____

_____

_____

_____

_____

_____

_____

_____

_____

_____

WHAT DID you do next? Think back to that time and try to recall what you did next. What, if anything, would you do differently?

_____

_____

_____

_____

_____

_____

_____

_____

_____

_____

_____

_____

_____

_____

WHAT WAS—or is—holding you back from moving forward on your path?

_____

_____

_____

_____

_____

_____

_____

_____

_____

_____

_____

_____

_____

_____

_____

_____

_____

_____

NOTES:

_____

_____

_____

_____

_____

_____

_____

_____

_____

_____

_____

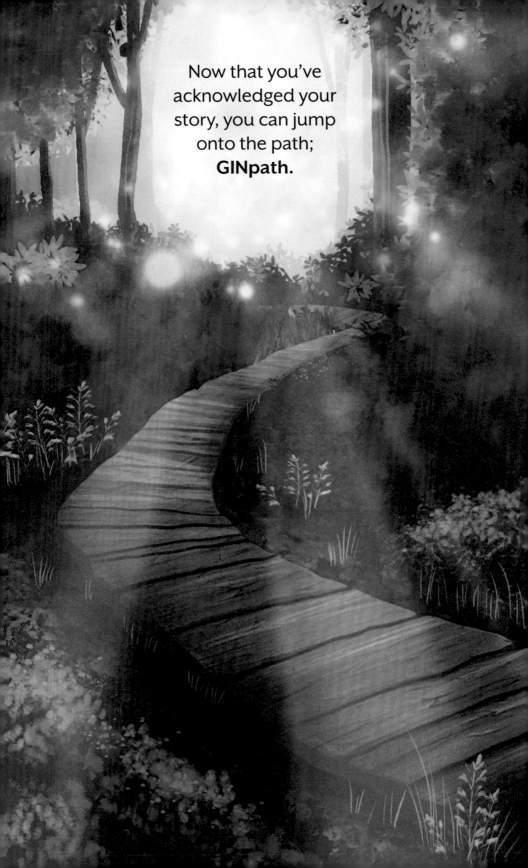

Now that you've acknowledged your story, you can jump onto the path; **GINpath.**

GINpath CONSISTS OF THREE MAIN COMPONENTS.

G̲ATHERING   I̲NTENTIONS   N̲URTURE

THESE THREE components will be broken down for you in the coming pages. This is the path that I walked down and walked through. I've continued on this path to get to where I am and I revisit it often. In fact, I visit and revisit parts of the path every day.

You can think of GINpath like a recipe. There are many different ingredients—you may want to use some of the ingredients exactly as suggested and you may want to swap some out for others.

Understand that the path is not linear and there will be twists, turns and obstacles along the way. The ingredients may change from day to day depending on what you need at different points on your path.

This journal is your guide and includes exercises, journal prompts, worksheets, tools and action steps that you can take to help you grow through these traumatic, adverse or difficult times and live the life you deserve. LET'S START ON YOUR PATH.

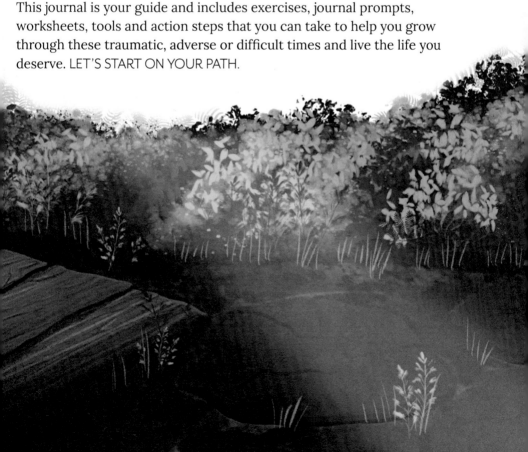

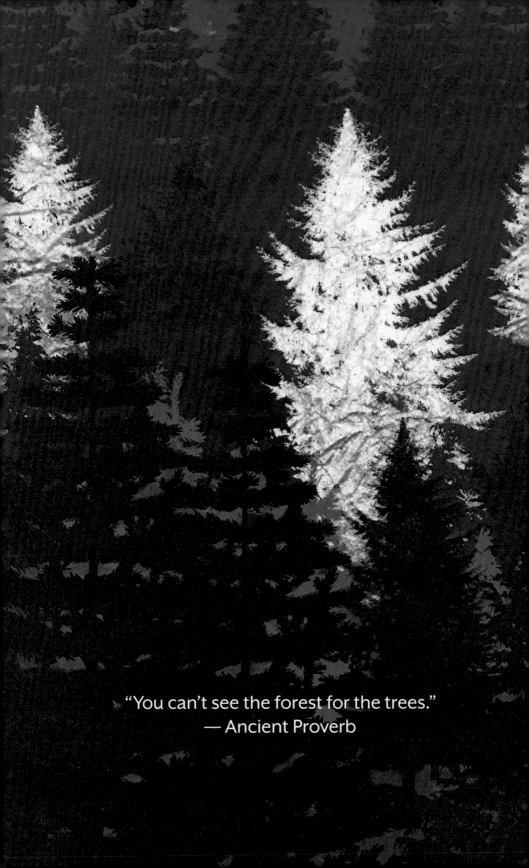

"You can't see the forest for the trees."
— Ancient Proverb

GATHERING

GATHERING

GATHERING WAS the first part of the path that I walked down. It was the process of understanding how I got here. I felt lost initially, as though I was standing alone in the middle of a forest and I didn't know how I got there or where I was going. I couldn't see the forest for the trees, as the ancient proverb says. I felt completely overwhelmed with the little details that I couldn't see the big picture. It was important to assess the situation at this phase. I needed to gather myself.

This is where the concept of Gathering was born. There were times when all I could do was gather my breath. Then, I gathered myself and my thoughts. The concept of gathering grew from there. I needed to start gathering information on the specific topics of my own traumatic experience.

I asked myself questions like, How did I get here? What happened? What is a narcissist? Would I ever love again? Do I know what unconditional love feels like?

What I began gathering were books, articles and journals. If reading isn't your thing, you could listen to podcasts.

If videos inspire you, resources like YouTube are helpful to begin gathering. You may utilize multiple forms of resources in your gathering process.

I gathered every form of information I could to better understand the path that led me to this place. I began reading, listening, watching and understanding. First, I focused externally on what was around me. I learned about my community and who was in it.

Then I began to take that next and difficult step and turned the lens inward to gather information about myself. I needed to truly discover myself again. I needed to break down the false armor I'd been carrying around and uncover and rediscover my own true identity. Gathering information can help you gain insight and perspective about your own circumstances.

This part of the path is designed to help you get curious and discover, or rediscover, things about yourself and your life to begin your journey of growing forward.

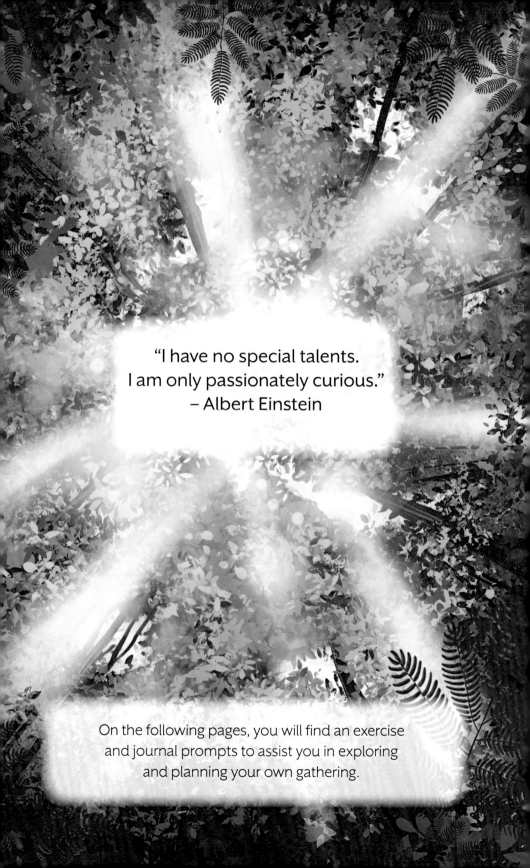

"I have no special talents.
I am only passionately curious."
– Albert Einstein

On the following pages, you will find an exercise
and journal prompts to assist you in exploring
and planning your own gathering.

BREATHE

WHEN YOU find yourself stuck, stressed or emotionally heightened, you can try a technique called box breathing to gather and recenter yourself. It's a simple practice and easy to learn. It can help you increase your concentration, bring you back to the moment and feel grounded so you can continue moving forward on your path. You can do this anywhere at any time. Box breathing can be done lying down or seated.

FOUR BASIC STEPS FOR BOX BREATHING, EACH LASTING FOUR SECONDS:

1. Breathe in slowly for a count of four. Feel the air fill your lungs.

2. Hold your breath for a count of four, trying not to inhale or exhale.

3. Slowly release your breath, exhaling through your mouth for four seconds.

4. Hold your breath for another four-count.

Repeat these steps until you feel as though you've gathered yourself.

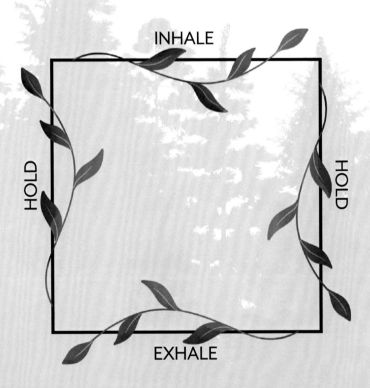

WHAT INFORMATION or categories of information would you like to gather about your story or situation to help you move forward on the path?

_____

_____

_____

_____

_____

_____

_____

_____

_____

_____

_____

_____

_____

_____

_____

_____

_____

_____

_____

_____

_____

_____

_____

_____

_____

_____

_____

_____

_____

RESEARCH AND make a list of resources that can help you gain a better understanding of what information you'd like to gather. Ideas for your list could include books, personal development courses, workshops, retreats, conferences, websites, blogs, newsletters, mentorship, articles, videos, podcasts, apps and more. Be sure to connect with me on Instagram (@ginnypriem) where I'll share a variety of resources.

-
-
-
-
-
-
-
-
-

KEY LEARNINGS FROM RESOURCES:

_____
_____
_____
_____
_____
_____
_____
_____

WHAT HAVE you discovered about yourself and your situation?

_____

_____

_____

_____

_____

_____

_____

_____

_____

WHAT ELSE would you like to gather and understand?

_____

_____

_____

_____

_____

_____

_____

_____

_____

WHAT'S NEXT on your path? Where would you like to go from here?

_____

_____

_____

_____

_____

_____

_____

_____

_____

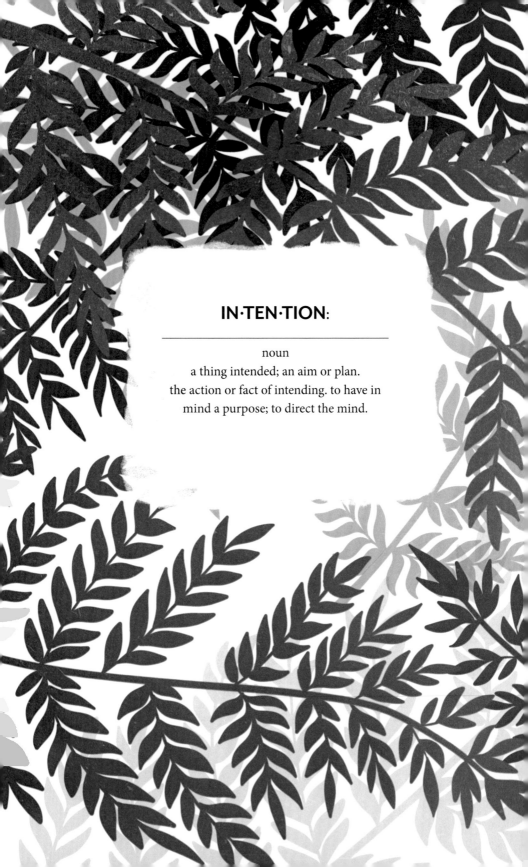

IN·TEN·TION:

noun
a thing intended; an aim or plan.
the action or fact of intending. to have in
mind a purpose; to direct the mind.

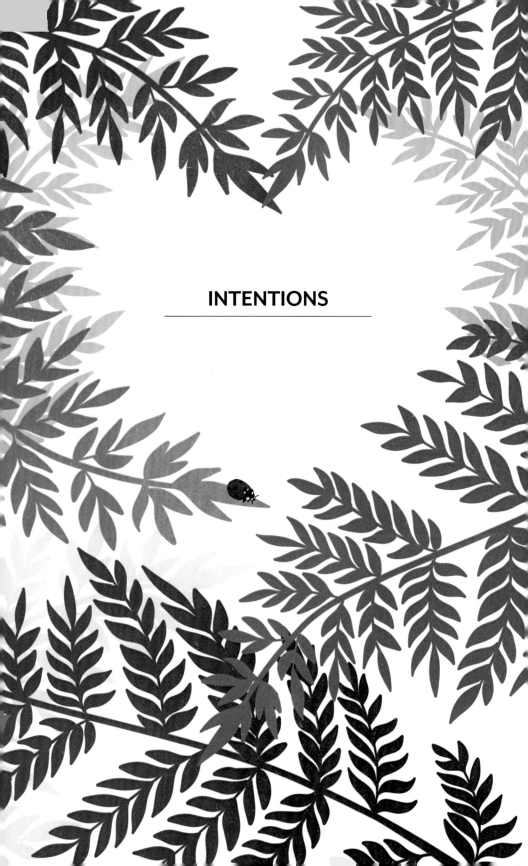

INTENTIONS

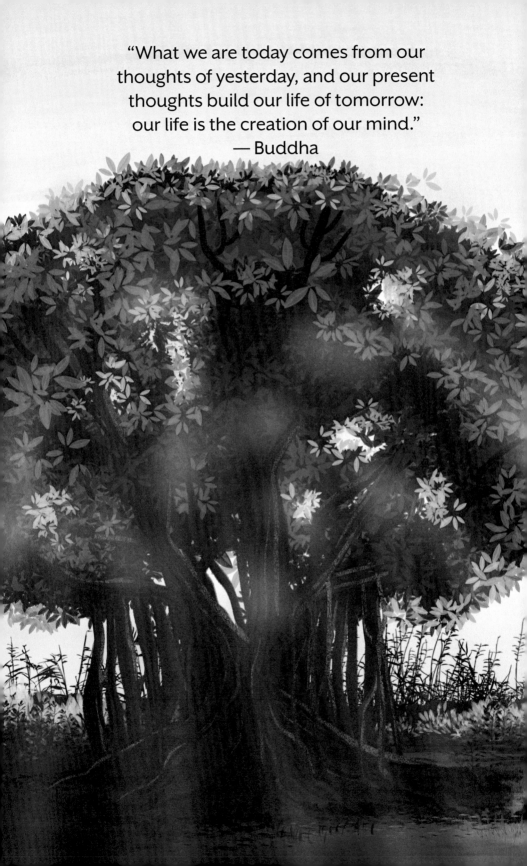

"What we are today comes from our thoughts of yesterday, and our present thoughts build our life of tomorrow: our life is the creation of our mind."
— Buddha

INTENTIONS

INTENTIONS NOT only help give us clarity to what we've gathered. They also help us get unstuck if we're stuck and help us start to see the clearing through the trees again. You've figured out where you are, and now there is a clear path of where you're going.

Intentions help you make that choice of where you're going and how you're moving forward. It's finding out what you want and what you don't want. This is where the path unfolds before you. Intentions for me are the mindfulness of what I do, what I think and what I say. In this section, you'll explore how your intentions can be the mindfulness of what you do, think and say.

On the following pages you'll find an exercise and journal prompts that can help bring awareness and intentionality to what you do, how you speak to and think about yourself. This space is for you to capture your thoughts and feelings.

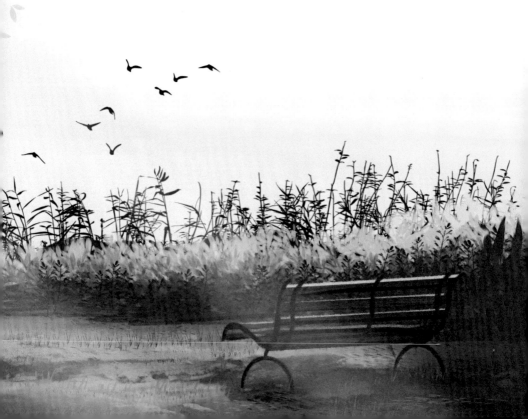

DO YOU engage in negative self-talk or hold a self-limiting belief you tell yourself or have told yourself in the past? If you're able, close your eyes and say this to yourself one time.

JOURNAL PROMPT: What did that bring up for you when you spoke to yourself in a negative way?

_____

_____

_____

_____

_____

_____

_____

_____

_____

Take that negative self-talk and flip the script. Try saying the opposite. If that doesn't feel possible right now, try something 10% kinder. Close your eyes again and say this kinder thought to yourself three times, maybe even with a smile on your face.

JOURNAL PROMPT: How do you feel speaking in a more kind, positive way to yourself?

_____

_____

_____

_____

_____

_____

_____

WHAT I learned on this part of the path is that it's not only what we do that's important. What we tell and think about ourselves also matters. The key with intentions is that this is where turning inward can lead to self-discovery and self-love. It's tough to expect others to be kind to you without being kind to yourself first.

Intentions can help to remove the need to seek external validation from others and help you become your most authentic self in order to shape your life into the one you deserve. Intentions can help you attract the life you're meant to have.

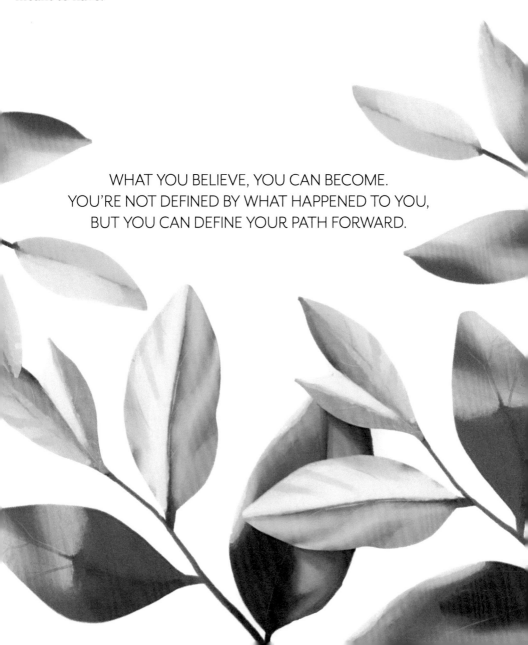

WHAT YOU BELIEVE, YOU CAN BECOME.
YOU'RE NOT DEFINED BY WHAT HAPPENED TO YOU,
BUT YOU CAN DEFINE YOUR PATH FORWARD.

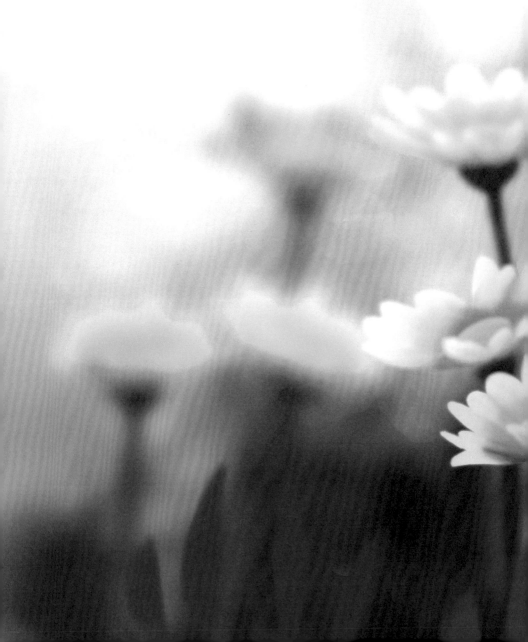

"Kindness starts with 'K'–
but it begins within."
— Ginny Priem

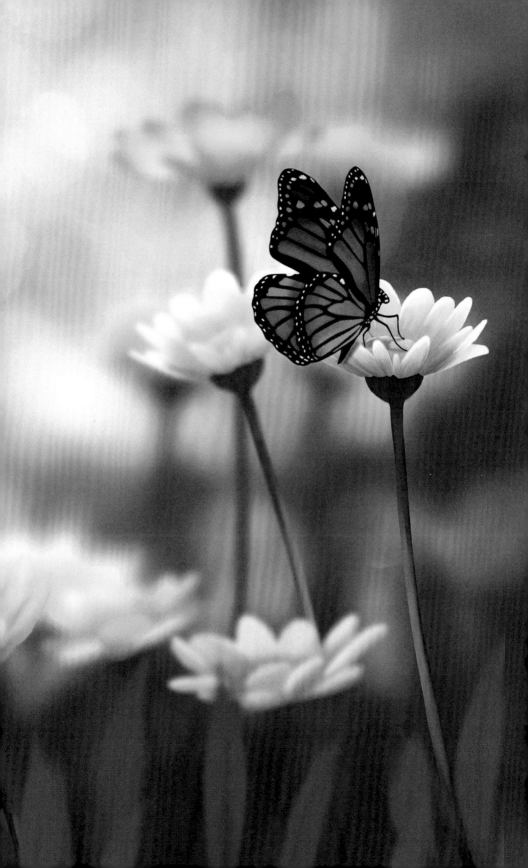

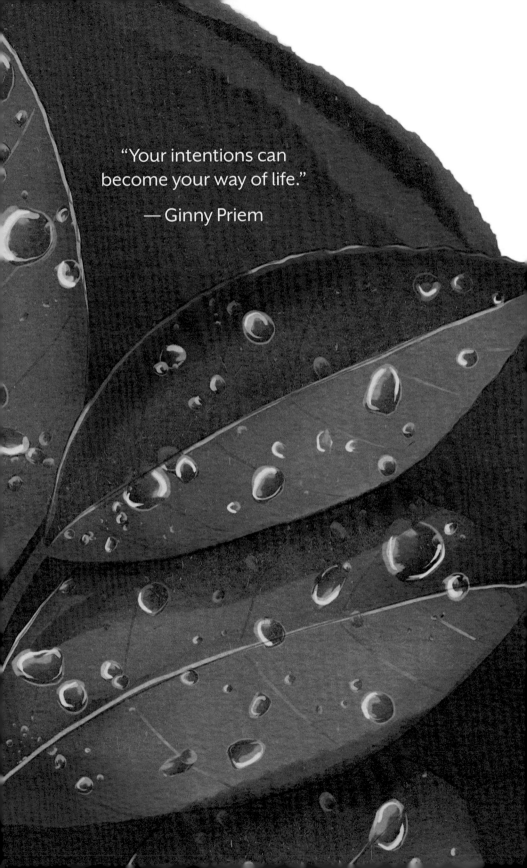

"Your intentions can
become your way of life."

— Ginny Priem

A HELPFUL study I gathered information from on my journey was by Dr. Masaru Emoto, a Japanese scientist. He studied the effects of human thoughts, words, sounds and intentions on water formations.

Water that was greeted with fearful and discordant thoughts, words and intentions formed disconnected, disfigured water crystals. In contrast, water that was greeted with compassionate and loving thoughts, words and intentions formed aesthetically pleasing snowflake designs and patterns.

If, on average, the human body is made up of approximately 60% water, imagine the transformation that's possible by purposefully cultivating our intentions.

Some people might think intentions are just a wish. They are much more than simply a dream if you revisit and place attention on them consistently. Intentions are also a place to express gratitude for where you are on your path so you can continue moving forward.

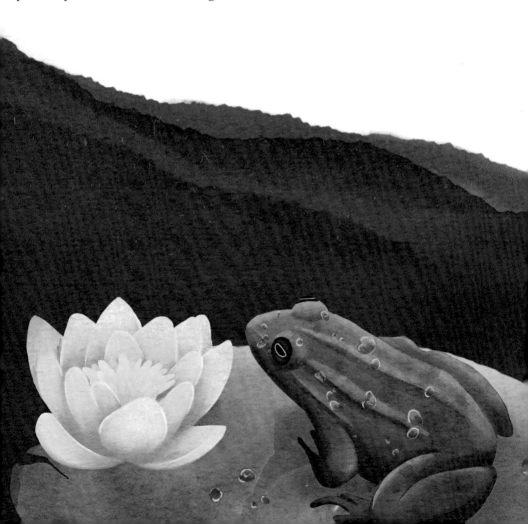

THINK ABOUT how your intentions or self-limiting thoughts have potentially been shaping your feelings and contributing to your overall happiness. What would you like to be intentional about that can bring you more peace and joy in your life?

_____

_____

_____

_____

_____

_____

_____

_____

_____

_____

WHAT DO you love about yourself or what are you learning to love?

_____

_____

_____

_____

_____

_____

_____

_____

_____

"The most successful people see adversity
not as a stumbling block, but as
a stepping-stone to greatness."
– Shawn Achor

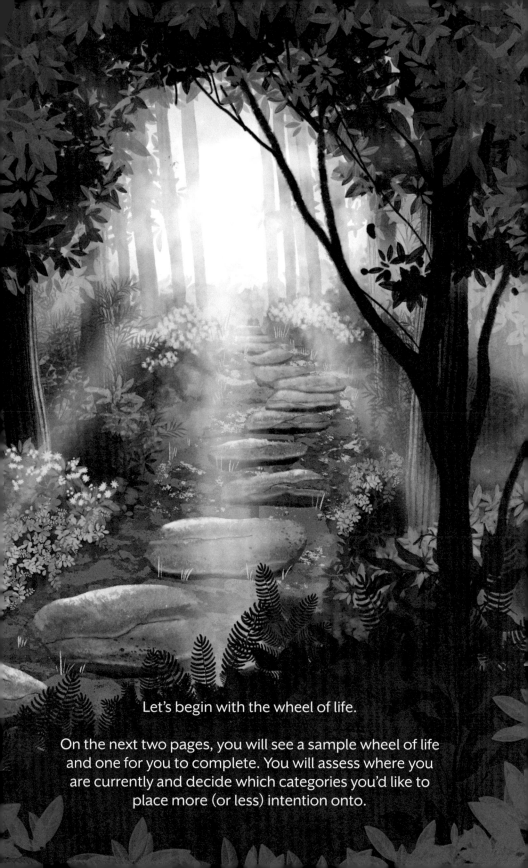

Let's begin with the wheel of life.

On the next two pages, you will see a sample wheel of life and one for you to complete. You will assess where you are currently and decide which categories you'd like to place more (or less) intention onto.

WHEEL OF LIFE

THE WHEEL OF LIFE is a great tool to help you improve your life balance. It helps you quickly and graphically identify and gather information on the areas in your life to which you want to devote more energy, and helps you understand where you might want to intentionally cut back.

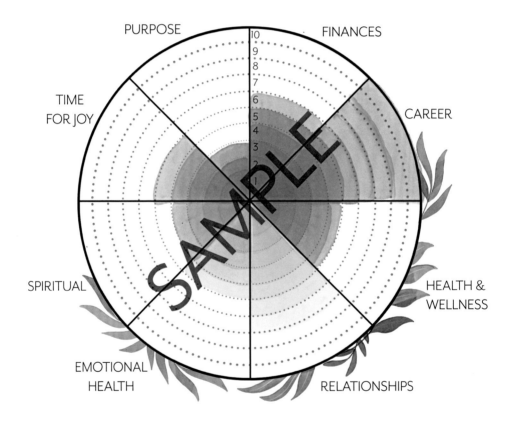

In the sample above, this person indicated that their highest level of mastery is in their career. In contrast, purpose represents their lowest category.

WHEEL OF LIFE

THE WHEEL OF LIFE is a great tool to help you improve your life balance. It helps you quickly and graphically identify and gather information on the areas in your life to which you want to devote more energy, and helps you understand where you might want to intentionally cut back.

Start at the tip of the pie piece and color out to where you believe represents your current level of mastery in each of the areas.

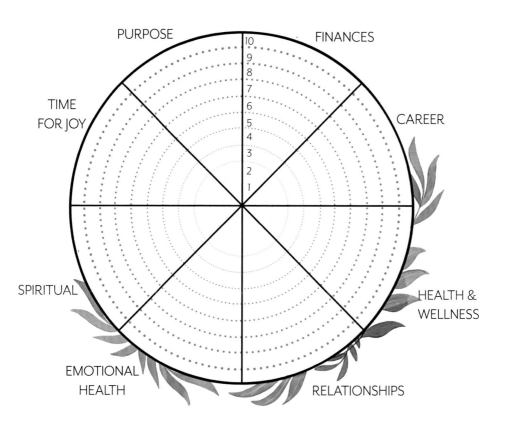

WHAT I'M proud of this month:

_____

_____

_____

_____

_____

NOW, TAKE those areas and think about what are some very specific things you'd like to be intentional about.

_____

_____

_____

_____

_____

_____

_____

_____

_____

_____

_____

_____

_____

_____

_____

_____

_____

_____

_____

HOW YOU express your intentions is key. Writing them in present tense helps attract, manifest and shape the life you want. For example, use statements that start with I AM rather than I hope or I will.

Your intentions can be as macro or as micro as you'd like them to be. Consider your wheel of life and what you envision for the categories you'd like to be intentional about.

If you're working on setting boundaries, a sample intention for this could be:

I honor my boundaries and only participate in the things I am comfortable with. My boundaries are respected by others.

It's important to be consistent with your intentions. In the back of this journal, you will find a full year of monthly pages to express your intentions. You can change them or keep them the same each month. I've kept some of the same intentions for years.

One method you could use as a guideline is the 3-6-9 method. This means that you will write and/or say your intentions three times in the morning, six times in the afternoon and nine times in the evening. Some believe this method helps attract what we give our attention to.

If you'd like to take it a step further, you could share your intentions with an accountability partner.

On the following page, you will find an intentions worksheet where you will write five positive intentions or affirmations that you will repeat throughout each day.

Get intentional with your first month of intentions!

INTENTIONS

INTENTION 1: _____
_____
_____
_____
_____

INTENTION 2: _____
_____
_____
_____
_____

INTENTION 3: _____
_____
_____
_____
_____

INTENTION 4: _____
_____
_____
_____
_____

INTENTION 5: _____
_____
_____
_____
_____

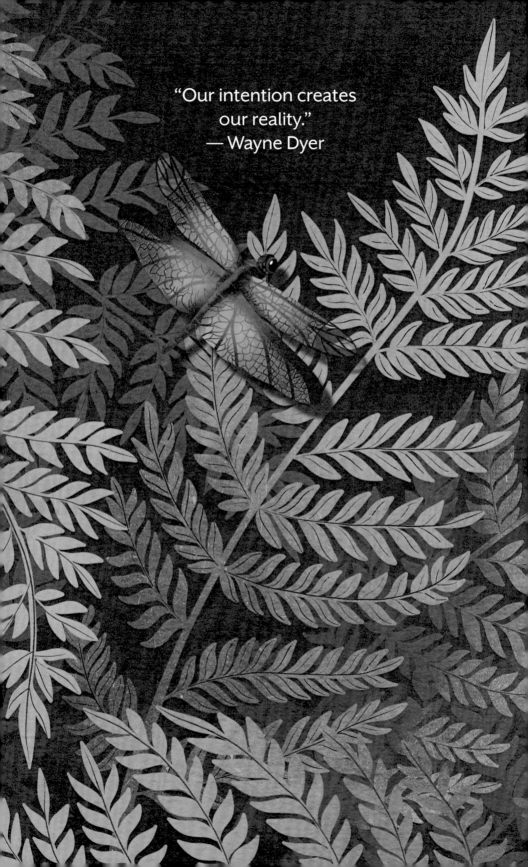

"Our intention creates
our reality."
— Wayne Dyer

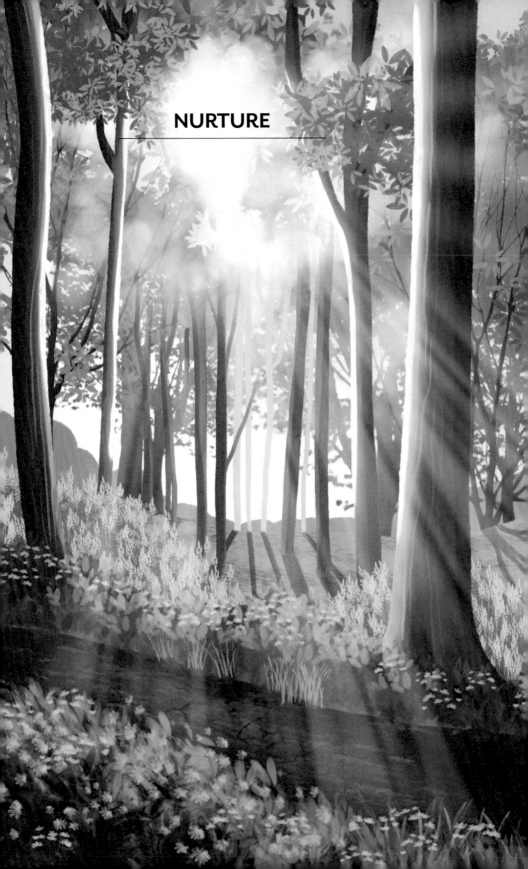

NURTURE

SO FAR, you've worked through gathering and understanding how you got here. You've gathered yourself and necessary information for you on your path. You've gathered your thoughts and your ideas. You got curious.

With intentions, you figured out where you're going.

You've arrived at the third part of GINpath: Nurture.

Some people view nurture as self-care. It includes self-care, but it's also much more. Nurture is all-encompassing. Often, people think about what they're putting in their bodies and how they care for themselves physically; working out and eating nutrient-dense foods. That is all part of nurture and so is taking care of yourself mentally and emotionally.

These are all important ingredients of the nurture component.

Since you know how you got here and where you're going, this is the "what's next." Nurture is not about going forward, but about *growing* forward.

When you're at the nurture phase, the path is illuminated. It gives you a clearer direction on where and how you're growing forward. Nurture encompasses physical, mental and emotional care and well-being.

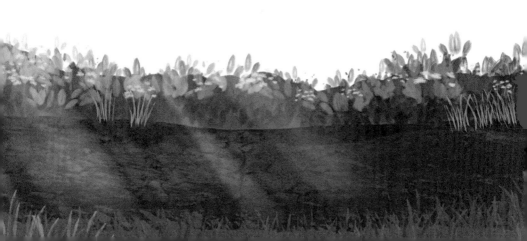

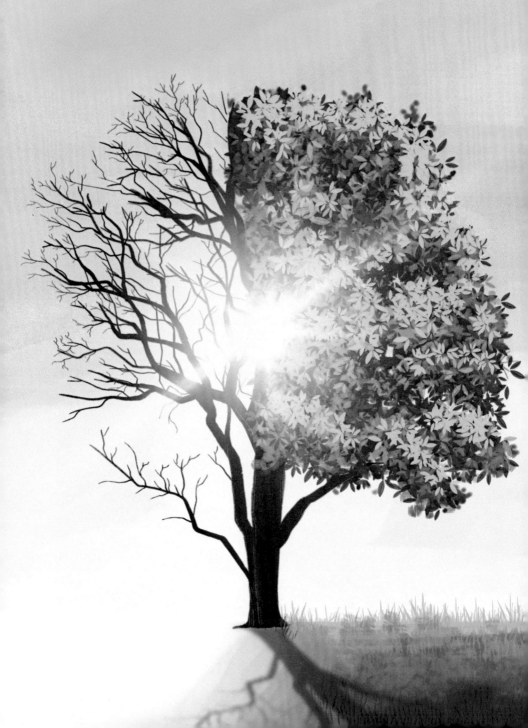

"Change is inevitable.
Transformation is by conscious choice."
— Heather Ash Amara

THERE ARE many different ways to nurture yourself. I personally discovered meditation. Consistently incorporating it into my routine changed my life. Nurture may look like prayer if faith is where you lean.

Yoga is a form of exercise where you can physically, mentally and emotionally nurture yourself. Being intentional about your nurture also matters. Yoga may be your choice for a good sweat or stretch. It may be that you need to sit within the four corners of your yoga mat to simply clear your mind.

There are many different forms of working out. Walking or running could be a way to physically move or mentally clear your mind. Lifting weights or high-intensity interval training are different ways to nurture yourself depending on what you're looking to get out of it.

Traditional therapy or coaching are other options to nurture yourself. Attending therapy sessions and finding a good coach or mentor have been successful strategies for many people.

Group support can be another way to nurture yourself when you're going through a traumatic situation or a time of adversity, and that ties back to the intention piece. If you're doing group support or some sort of group therapy, being intentional about the type of group it is and who's in it can play a part in what you get out of it.

Nurture could look like getting a manicure, pedicure, massage or facial. If that isn't doable, taking 10 minutes of quiet time can be a suitable option. You may enroll in a personal development course, attend a retreat or a conference or even take a vacation.

In addition to journaling here, creating a vision board is another option to place intention on how you nurture yourself.

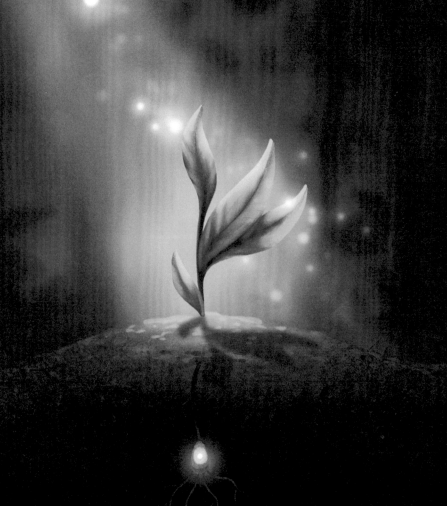

"In those traumatic, difficult, dark times, it may feel like you're a seed buried deep beneath the earth. Consider this: have you actually been planted?"
— Ginny Priem

WHEN YOU are in this growing phase and nurturing yourself, think about planting seeds or trees for your future. Nurture is how you water it and care for it to grow. Think about what that looks like for you. You can always relate that back to intentions. Consider where you're going and then water it and nurture it to care for yourself by asking, "How am I growing forward?"

Nurturing is more than just the foods that you're consuming and the nutrients that you're putting in your body. Think about the books and the social media you're consuming. This is different from gathering information and reading books. This is more about what you might be unconsciously consuming.

Consider how what you're unconsciously consuming might be impacting your mood. Think about what you're eating, how you're moving, what you're watching on social media and TV. How is this content impacting your life? It's important to choose what you're nurturing and be mindful about how you're incorporating these things into your path forward.

NOTES:
_____
_____
_____
_____
_____
_____
_____
_____
_____
_____
_____
_____

WHAT IS important for you to nurture and protect for your physical, mental and emotional well-being?

_____

_____

_____

_____

_____

_____

_____

_____

_____

_____

_____

_____

_____

_____

_____

_____

_____

_____

_____

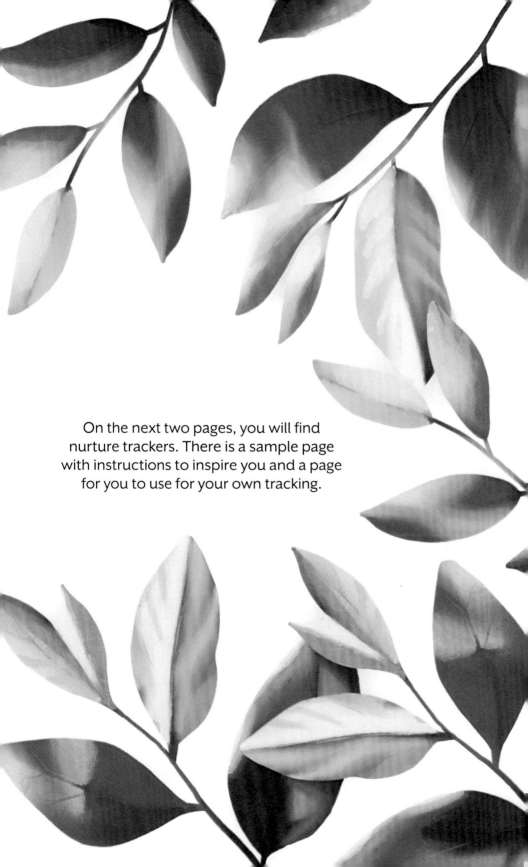

On the next two pages, you will find
nurture trackers. There is a sample page
with instructions to inspire you and a page
for you to use for your own tracking.

NURTURE TRACKER

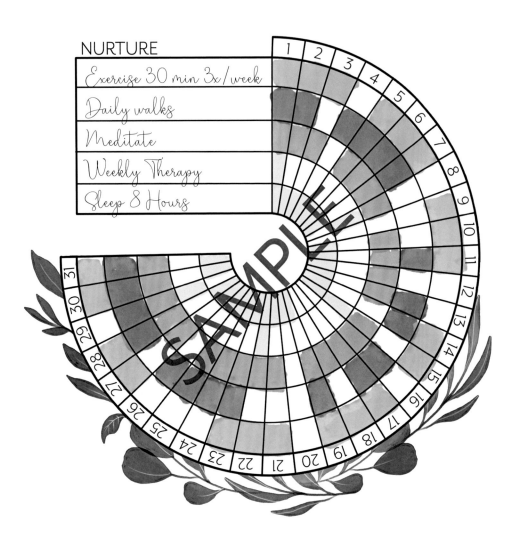

NURTURE

| Exercise 30 min 3x/week |
| Daily walks |
| Meditate |
| Weekly Therapy |
| Sleep 8 Hours |

THIS TOOL is provided to assist you in tracking the ways you nurture yourself. There is a space to fill in for each day of the month you accomplish what you aimed to nurture. Visit this regularly, even daily, to help create healthy habits.

NURTURE TRACKER

NURTURE

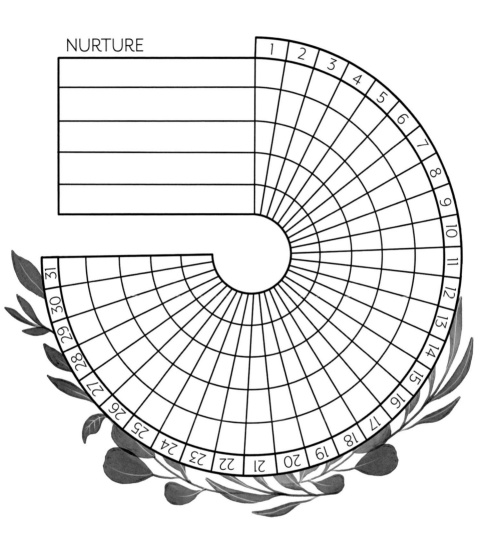

WHAT I'M proud of this month:

_____

_____

_____

_____

_____

_____

EMOTIONAL VIBRATION CHART

THIS IMAGE, based on the emotional vibration chart, is a tool designed to help you identify which emotions produce higher frequencies and which produce lower frequencies. The goal is to use this as a reference and track your progress of moving toward a state of consistently higher vibrations.

Contemplate the emotions you've been feeling recently. On the chart, circle the emotions that most closely depict how you've felt over the past month or so.

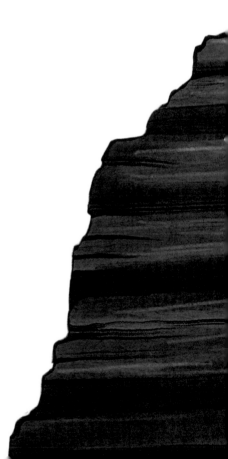

ENLIGHTENMENT

PEACE

JOY

LOVE

REASON

ACCEPTANCE

WILLINGNESS

NEUTRALITY

COURAGE

PRIDE

ANGER

DESIRE

FEAR

GRIEF

APATHY

GUILT

SHAME

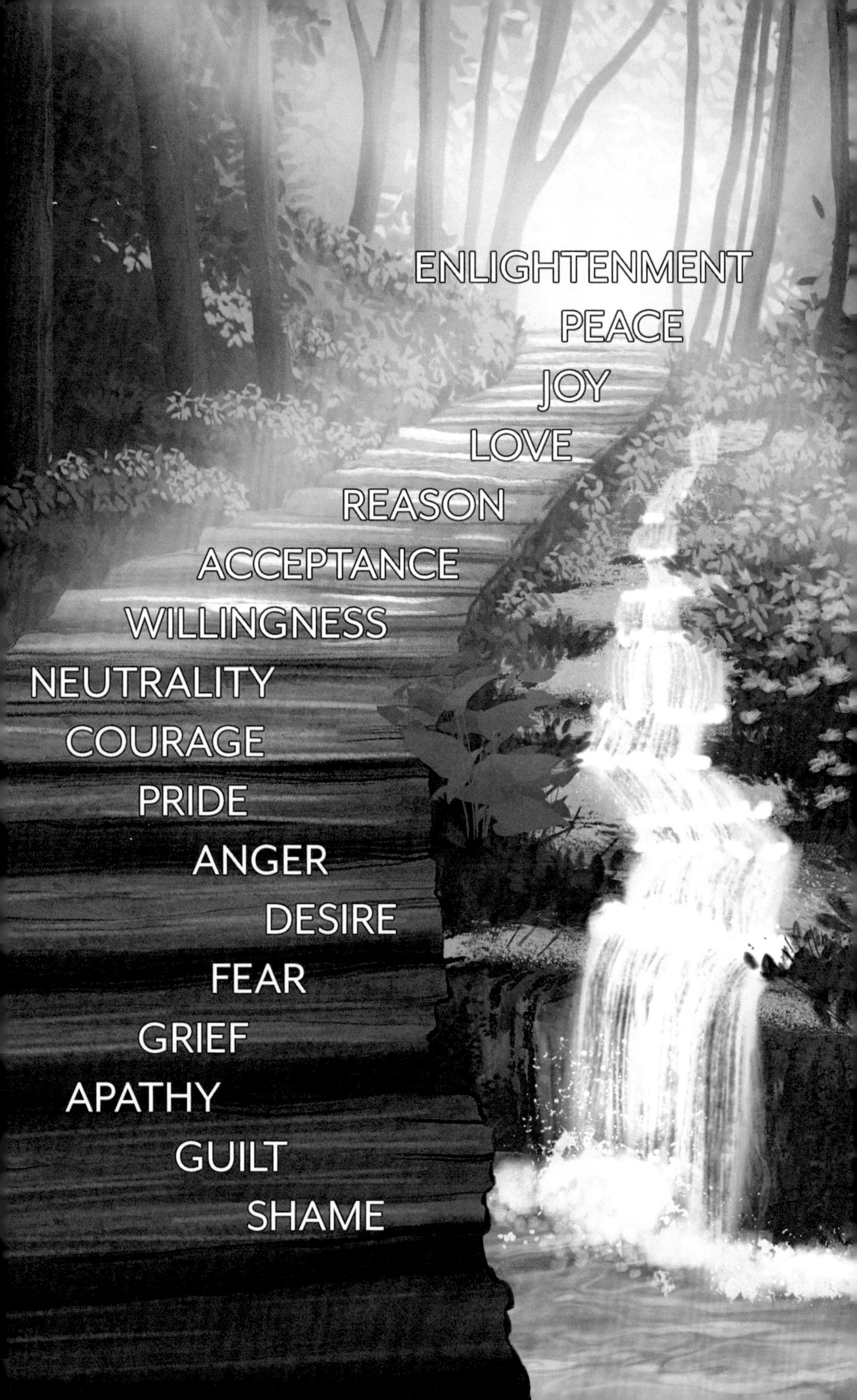

ENLIGHTENMENT
PEACE
JOY
LOVE
REASON
ACCEPTANCE
WILLINGNESS
NEUTRALITY
COURAGE
PRIDE
ANGER
DESIRE
FEAR
GRIEF
APATHY
GUILT
SHAME

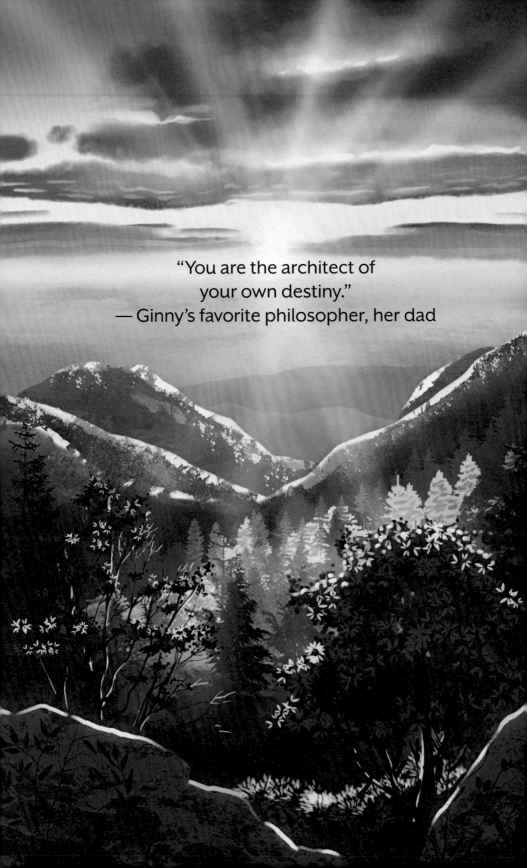

"You are the architect of
your own destiny."
— Ginny's favorite philosopher, her dad

GINpath WAS my way of processing and working through my experience to discover myself and find self-love. These are the tools that helped, and continue to help, me be the best and most authentic version of myself. And now it's your path. It's important to remember that there's no stopwatch or time frame on your healing and growing journey. Your pace may vary and the components on the path may interweave while you continue growing forward.

You know you're making progress when you tell your story differently. These three components—Gathering, Intentions and Nurture—are what helped me tell my story differently.

GINpath helped me with overcoming what's mine. Now that it's your path, it can help you overcome what's yours and continue on your bright journey ahead.

On the following pages, you will find an additional 12 full months of the worksheets and journal prompts you've already completed in this journal. These are designed to help you stay on your path forward and to be better equipped with tools to face difficult situations that come your way.

If you'd like to see examples for any of the journal pages, make sure you connect with me on social media (@ginnypriem) and visit my website (www.ginnypriem.com) where I'll be sharing samples from *I'm My Favorite*.

LET'S GET GROWING!

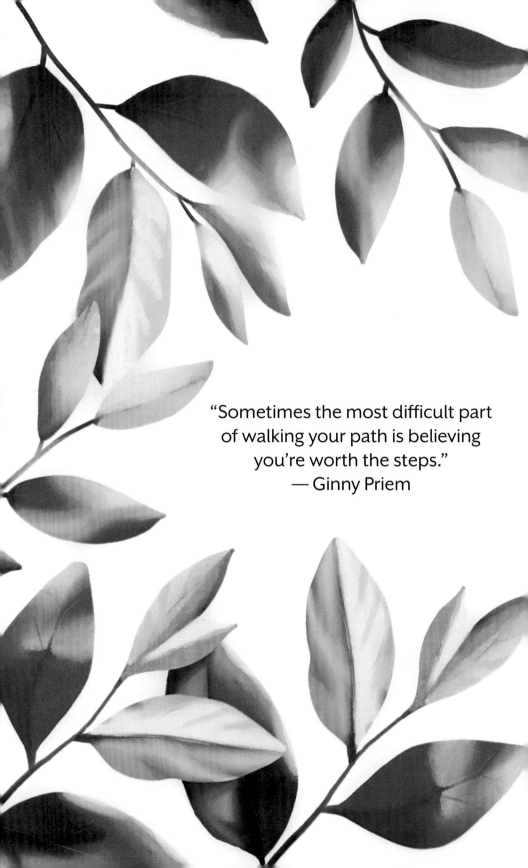

"Sometimes the most difficult part of walking your path is believing you're worth the steps."
— Ginny Priem

MONTH:

_____

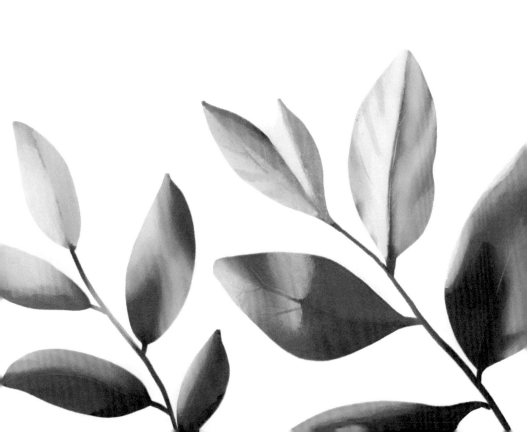

WHAT IS the situation or circumstances that put you in the face of adversity, a traumatic time or difficult experience? This may include —but is not limited to— physical injury, illness, loss, financial issues, mental strain or emotional harm. What's your story?

_____

_____

_____

_____

_____

_____

_____

_____

_____

_____

_____

_____

_____

_____

_____

_____

_____

_____

_____

_____

_____

_____

_____

_____

_____

_____

_____

_____

USE THIS space to capture additional details about where you were, what you were doing and how this impacted your life. What other contributing factors or people were involved?

_____
_____
_____
_____
_____
_____
_____
_____
_____
_____
_____

WHAT WAS your mindset at the time? Use this area to jot down the feelings you processed. Did you feel fear, anger, frustration, overwhelm, devastation, disbelief or optimism? What feelings are coming up for you now about your story?

_____
_____
_____
_____
_____
_____
_____
_____
_____
_____
_____
_____
_____

WHAT DID you do next? Think back to that time and try to recall what you did next. What, if anything, would you do differently?

_____

_____

_____

_____

_____

_____

_____

_____

_____

_____

_____

_____

WHAT WAS—or is—holding you back from moving forward on your path?

_____

_____

_____

_____

_____

_____

_____

_____

_____

_____

_____

_____

_____

BREATHE

WHEN YOU find yourself stuck, stressed or emotionally heightened, you can try a technique called box breathing to gather and recenter yourself. It's a simple practice and easy to learn. It can help you increase your concentration, bring you back to the moment and feel grounded so you can continue moving forward on your path. You can do this anywhere at any time. Box breathing can be done lying down or seated.

FOUR BASIC STEPS FOR BOX BREATHING, EACH LASTING FOUR SECONDS:

1. Breathe in slowly for a count of four. Feel the air fill your lungs.

2. Hold your breath for a count of four, trying not to inhale or exhale.

3. Slowly release your breath, exhaling through your mouth for four seconds.

4. Hold your breath for another four-count.

Repeat these steps until you feel as though you've gathered yourself.

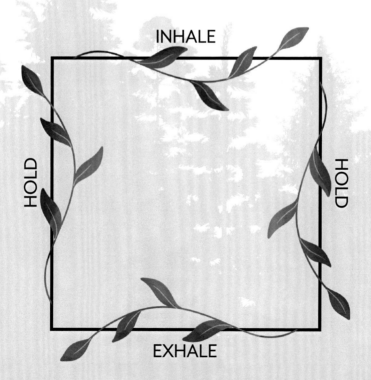

RESEARCH AND make a list of resources that can help you gain a better understanding of what information you'd like to gather. Ideas for your list could include books, personal development courses, workshops, retreats, conferences, websites, blogs, newsletters, mentorship, articles, videos, podcasts, apps and more. Be sure to connect with me on Instagram (@ginnypriem) where I'll share a variety of resources.

-
-
-
-
-
-
-
-
-
-

KEY LEARNINGS FROM RESOURCES:

_____

_____

_____

_____

_____

_____

_____

_____

_____

WHAT HAVE you discovered about yourself and your situation?

_____

_____

_____

_____

_____

_____

_____

_____

WHAT ELSE would you like to gather and understand?

_____

_____

_____

_____

_____

_____

_____

WHAT'S NEXT on your path? Where would you like to go from here?

_____

_____

_____

_____

_____

_____

_____

_____

DO YOU engage in negative self-talk or hold a self-limiting belief you tell yourself or have told yourself in the past? If you're able, close your eyes and say this to yourself one time.

JOURNAL PROMPT: What did that bring up for you when you spoke to yourself in a negative way?

_____

_____

_____

_____

_____

_____

_____

_____

_____

Take that negative self-talk and flip the script. Try saying the opposite. If that doesn't feel possible right now, try something 10% kinder. Close your eyes again and say this kinder thought to yourself three times, maybe even with a smile on your face.

JOURNAL PROMPT: How do you feel speaking in a more kind, positive way to yourself?

_____

_____

_____

_____

_____

_____

_____

THINK ABOUT how your intentions or self-limiting thoughts have potentially been shaping your feelings and contributing to your overall happiness. What would you like to be intentional about that can bring you more peace and joy in your life?

_____

_____

_____

_____

_____

_____

_____

_____

_____

_____

What you believe, you can become.
You're not defined by what happened to you,
but you can define your path forward.

WHAT DO you love about yourself or what are you learning to love?

_____

_____

_____

_____

_____

_____

_____

_____

_____

_____

WHEEL OF LIFE

THE WHEEL OF LIFE is a great tool to help you improve your life balance. It helps you quickly and graphically identify and gather information on the areas in your life to which you want to devote more energy, and helps you understand where you might want to intentionally cut back.

Start at the tip of the pie piece and color out to where you believe represents your current level of mastery in each of the areas.

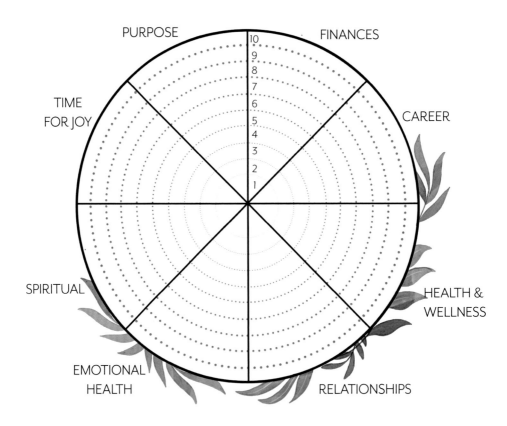

WHAT I'M proud of this month:

_____

_____

_____

_____

_____

INTENTIONS

INTENTION 1: _____

_____

_____

_____

_____

INTENTION 2: _____

_____

_____

_____

_____

INTENTION 3: _____

_____

_____

_____

_____

INTENTION 4: _____

_____

_____

_____

_____

INTENTION 5: _____

_____

_____

_____

_____

EMOTIONAL VIBRATION CHART

CONTEMPLATE THE emotions you've been feeling recently. On the chart, circle the emotions that most closely depict how you've felt over the past month or so.

ENLIGHTENMENT

PEACE

JOY

LOVE

REASON

ACCEPTANCE

WILLINGNESS

NEUTRALITY

COURAGE

PRIDE

ANGER

DESIRE

FEAR

GRIEF

APATHY

GUILT

SHAME

NOTES:

NURTURE TRACKER

NURTURE

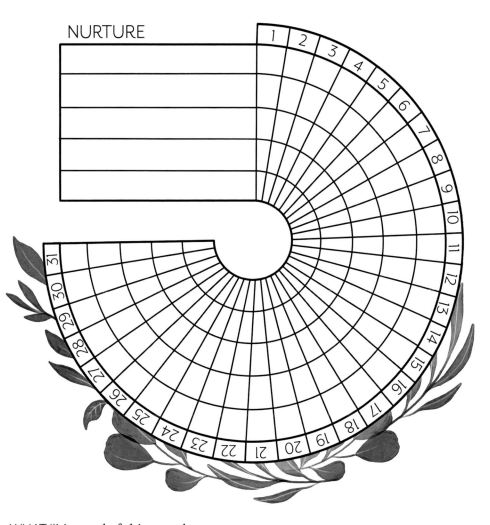

WHAT I'M proud of this month:

_____
_____
_____
_____
_____
_____
_____

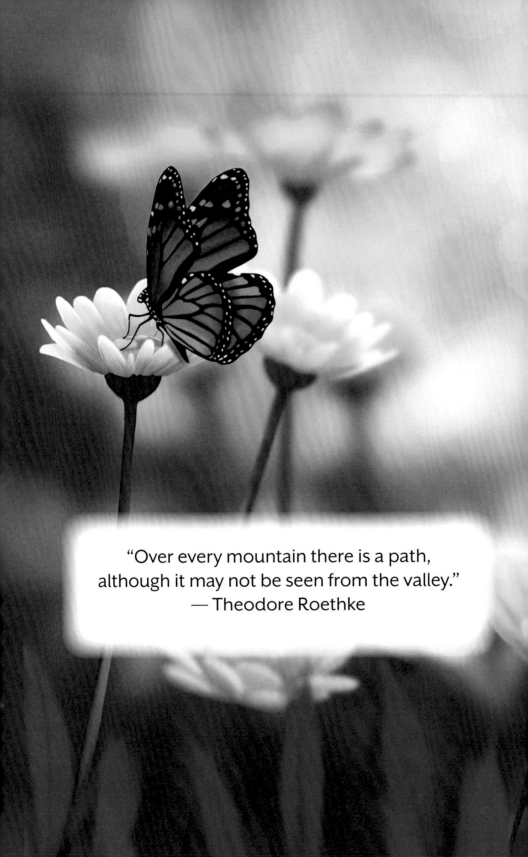

"Over every mountain there is a path,
although it may not be seen from the valley."
— Theodore Roethke

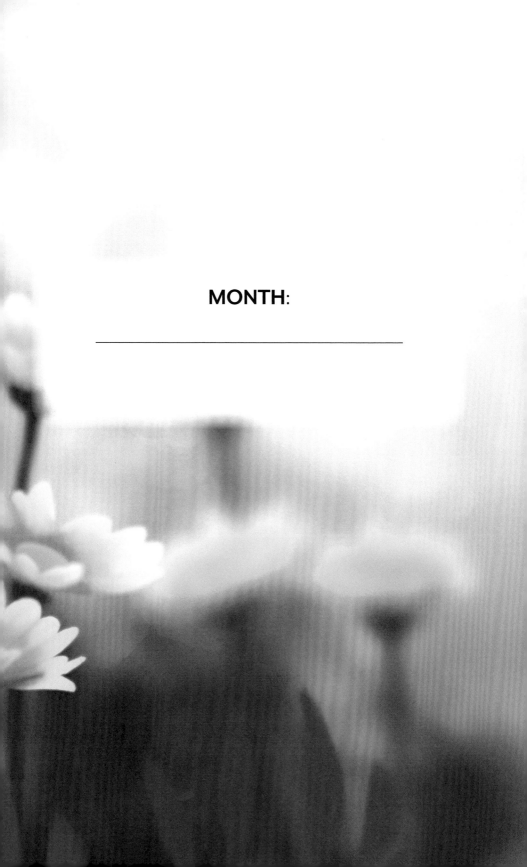

MONTH:

_____

WHAT IS the situation or circumstances that put you in the face of adversity, a traumatic time or difficult experience? This may include —but is not limited to— physical injury, illness, loss, financial issues, mental strain or emotional harm. What's your story?

_____

_____

_____

_____

_____

_____

_____

_____

_____

_____

_____

_____

_____

_____

_____

_____

_____

_____

_____

_____

_____

_____

_____

_____

_____

_____

_____

_____

USE THIS space to capture additional details about where you were, what you were doing and how this impacted your life. What other contributing factors or people were involved?

_____

_____

_____

_____

_____

_____

_____

_____

_____

_____

_____

WHAT WAS your mindset at the time? Use this area to jot down the feelings you processed. Did you feel fear, anger, frustration, overwhelm, devastation, disbelief or optimism? What feelings are coming up for you now about your story?

_____

_____

_____

_____

_____

_____

_____

_____

_____

_____

_____

_____

_____

_____

WHAT DID you do next? Think back to that time and try to recall what you did next. What, if anything, would you do differently?

_____

_____

_____

_____

_____

_____

_____

_____

_____

_____

_____

_____

_____

WHAT WAS—or is—holding you back from moving forward on your path?

_____

_____

_____

_____

_____

_____

_____

_____

_____

_____

_____

_____

_____

BREATHE

WHEN YOU find yourself stuck, stressed or emotionally heightened, you can try a technique called box breathing to gather and recenter yourself. It's a simple practice and easy to learn. It can help you increase your concentration, bring you back to the moment and feel grounded so you can continue moving forward on your path. You can do this anywhere at any time. Box breathing can be done lying down or seated.

FOUR BASIC STEPS FOR BOX BREATHING, EACH LASTING FOUR SECONDS:

1. Breathe in slowly for a count of four. Feel the air fill your lungs.

2. Hold your breath for a count of four, trying not to inhale or exhale.

3. Slowly release your breath, exhaling through your mouth for four seconds.

4. Hold your breath for another four-count.

Repeat these steps until you feel as though you've gathered yourself.

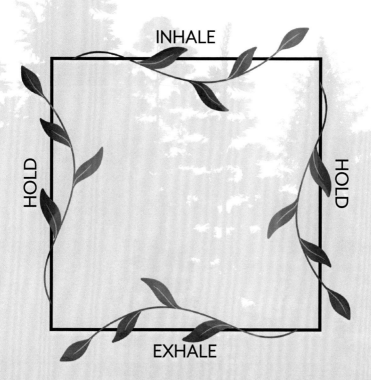

RESEARCH AND make a list of resources that can help you gain a better understanding of what information you'd like to gather. Ideas for your list could include books, personal development courses, workshops, retreats, conferences, websites, blogs, newsletters, mentorship, articles, videos, podcasts, apps and more. Be sure to connect with me on Instagram (@ginnypriem) where I'll share a variety of resources.

-
-
-
-
-
-
-
-
-

KEY LEARNINGS FROM RESOURCES:

_____
_____
_____
_____
_____
_____
_____
_____

WHAT HAVE you discovered about yourself and your situation?

_____
_____
_____
_____
_____
_____
_____
_____
_____

WHAT ELSE would you like to gather and understand?

_____
_____
_____
_____
_____
_____
_____
_____
_____

WHAT'S NEXT on your path? Where would you like to go from here?

_____
_____
_____
_____
_____
_____
_____
_____
_____

DO YOU engage in negative self-talk or hold a self-limiting belief you tell yourself or have told yourself in the past? If you're able, close your eyes and say this to yourself one time.

JOURNAL PROMPT: What did that bring up for you when you spoke to yourself in a negative way?

_____

_____

_____

_____

_____

_____

_____

_____

_____

Take that negative self-talk and flip the script. Try saying the opposite. If that doesn't feel possible right now, try something 10% kinder. Close your eyes again and say this kinder thought to yourself three times, maybe even with a smile on your face.

JOURNAL PROMPT: How do you feel speaking in a more kind, positive way to yourself?

_____

_____

_____

_____

_____

_____

_____

THINK ABOUT how your intentions or self-limiting thoughts have potentially been shaping your feelings and contributing to your overall happiness. What would you like to be intentional about that can bring you more peace and joy in your life?

_____

_____

_____

_____

_____

_____

_____

_____

_____

_____

_____

What you believe, you can become.
You're not defined by what happened to you,
but you can define your path forward.

WHAT DO you love about yourself or what are you learning to love?

_____

_____

_____

_____

_____

_____

_____

_____

_____

_____

WHEEL OF LIFE

THE WHEEL OF LIFE is a great tool to help you improve your life balance. It helps you quickly and graphically identify and gather information on the areas in your life to which you want to devote more energy, and helps you understand where you might want to intentionally cut back.

Start at the tip of the pie piece and color out to where you believe represents your current level of mastery in each of the areas.

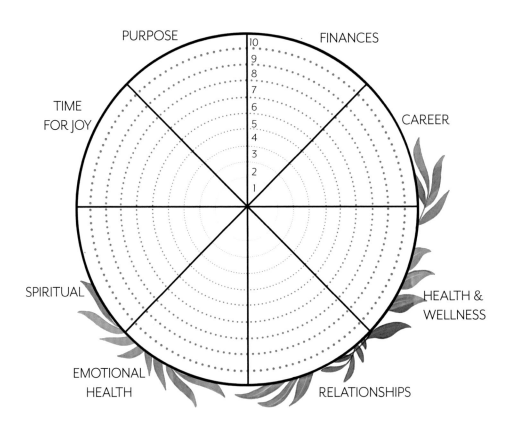

WHAT I'M proud of this month:

_____

_____

_____

_____

_____

INTENTIONS

INTENTION 1: _____
_____
_____
_____
_____

INTENTION 2: _____
_____
_____
_____
_____

INTENTION 3: _____
_____
_____
_____
_____

INTENTION 4: _____
_____
_____
_____
_____

INTENTION 5: _____
_____
_____
_____
_____

EMOTIONAL VIBRATION CHART

CONTEMPLATE THE emotions you've been feeling recently. On the chart, circle the emotions that most closely depict how you've felt over the past month or so.

ENLIGHTENMENT

PEACE

JOY

LOVE

REASON

ACCEPTANCE

WILLINGNESS

NEUTRALITY

COURAGE

PRIDE

ANGER

DESIRE

FEAR

GRIEF

APATHY

GUILT

SHAME

NOTES:

_____
_____
_____
_____
_____
_____
_____
_____
_____
_____
_____
_____
_____
_____
_____
_____
_____
_____
_____
_____

NURTURE TRACKER

NURTURE

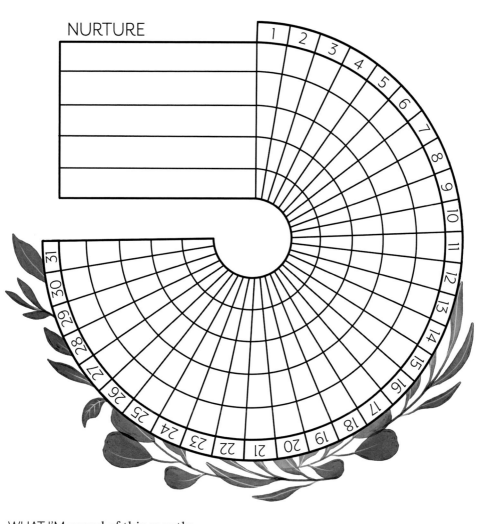

WHAT I'M proud of this month:

_____
_____
_____
_____
_____
_____
_____

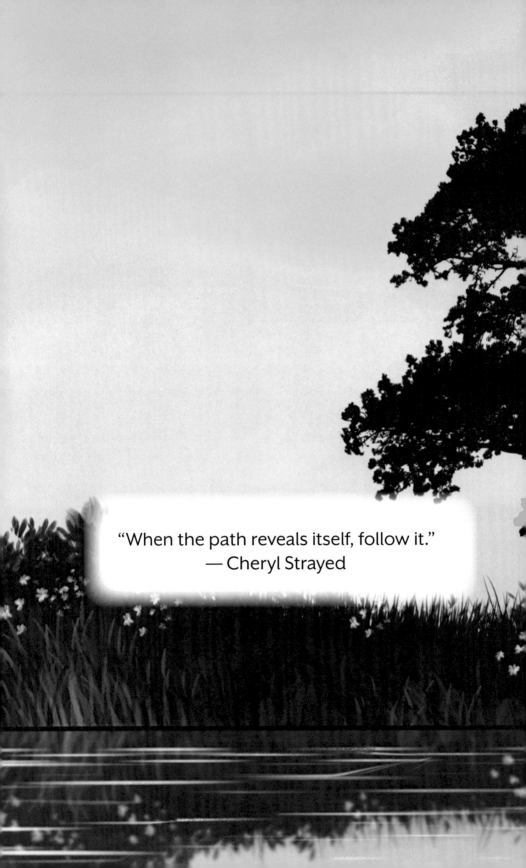

"When the path reveals itself, follow it."
— Cheryl Strayed

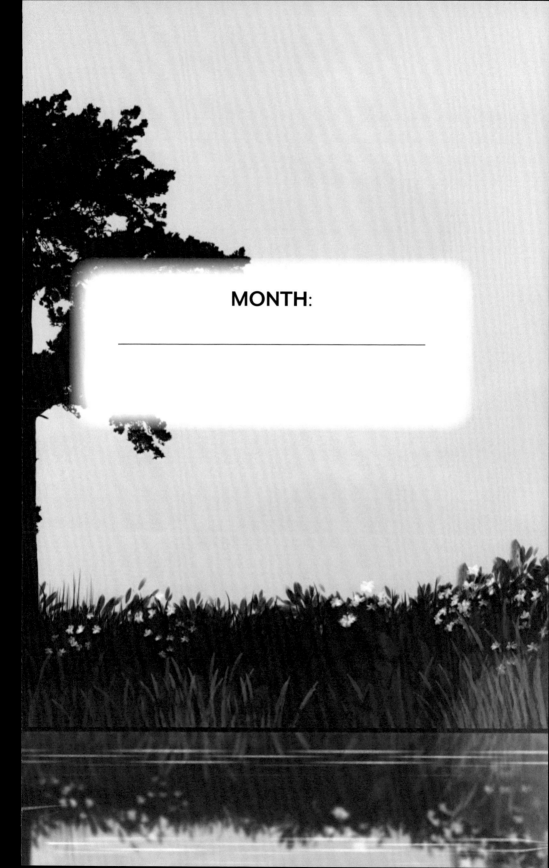

MONTH:

WHAT IS the situation or circumstances that put you in the face of adversity, a traumatic time or difficult experience? This may include —but is not limited to   physical injury, illness, loss, financial issues, mental strain or emotional harm. What's your story?

_____

_____

_____

_____

_____

_____

_____

_____

_____

_____

_____

_____

_____

_____

_____

_____

_____

_____

_____

_____

_____

_____

_____

_____

_____

_____

_____

_____

_____

_____

USE THIS space to capture additional details about where you were, what you were doing and how this impacted your life. What other contributing factors or people were involved?

_____

_____

_____

_____

_____

_____

_____

_____

_____

_____

_____

WHAT WAS your mindset at the time? Use this area to jot down the feelings you processed. Did you feel fear, anger, frustration, overwhelm, devastation, disbelief or optimism? What feelings are coming up for you now about your story?

_____

_____

_____

_____

_____

_____

_____

_____

_____

_____

_____

_____

_____

_____

WHAT DID you do next? Think back to that time and try to recall what you did next. What, if anything, would you do differently?

_____

_____

_____

_____

_____

_____

_____

_____

_____

_____

_____

_____

_____

WHAT WAS—or is—holding you back from moving forward on your path?

_____

_____

_____

_____

_____

_____

_____

_____

_____

_____

_____

_____

_____

_____

BREATHE

WHEN YOU find yourself stuck, stressed or emotionally heightened, you can try a technique called box breathing to gather and recenter yourself. It's a simple practice and easy to learn. It can help you increase your concentration, bring you back to the moment and feel grounded so you can continue moving forward on your path. You can do this anywhere at any time. Box breathing can be done lying down or seated.

FOUR BASIC STEPS FOR BOX BREATHING, EACH LASTING FOUR SECONDS:

1. Breathe in slowly for a count of four. Feel the air fill your lungs.

2. Hold your breath for a count of four, trying not to inhale or exhale.

3. Slowly release your breath, exhaling through your mouth for four seconds.

4. Hold your breath for another four-count.

Repeat these steps until you feel as though you've gathered yourself.

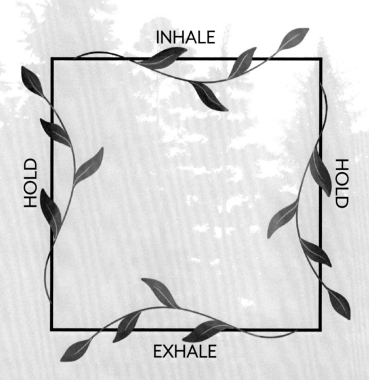

RESEARCH AND make a list of resources that can help you gain a better understanding of what information you'd like to gather. Ideas for your list could include books, personal development courses, workshops, retreats, conferences, websites, blogs, newsletters, mentorship, articles, videos, podcasts, apps and more. Be sure to connect with me on Instagram (@ginnypriem) where I'll share a variety of resources.

-
-
-
-
-
-
-
-
-
-

KEY LEARNINGS FROM RESOURCES:

_____

_____

_____

_____

_____

_____

_____

_____

WHAT HAVE you discovered about yourself and your situation?

_____

_____

_____

_____

_____

_____

_____

_____

_____

WHAT ELSE would you like to gather and understand?

_____

_____

_____

_____

_____

_____

_____

_____

_____

WHAT'S NEXT on your path? Where would you like to go from here?

_____

_____

_____

_____

_____

_____

_____

_____

_____

DO YOU engage in negative self-talk or hold a self-limiting belief you tell yourself or have told yourself in the past? If you're able, close your eyes and say this to yourself one time.

JOURNAL PROMPT: What did that bring up for you when you spoke to yourself in a negative way?

_____

_____

_____

_____

_____

_____

_____

_____

_____

Take that negative self-talk and flip the script. Try saying the opposite. If that doesn't feel possible right now, try something 10% kinder. Close your eyes again and say this kinder thought to yourself three times, maybe even with a smile on your face.

JOURNAL PROMPT: How do you feel speaking in a more kind, positive way to yourself?

_____

_____

_____

_____

_____

_____

_____

THINK ABOUT how your intentions or self-limiting thoughts have potentially been shaping your feelings and contributing to your overall happiness. What would you like to be intentional about that can bring you more peace and joy in your life?

_____

_____

_____

_____

_____

_____

_____

_____

_____

_____

_____

What you believe, you can become.
You're not defined by what happened to you,
but you can define your path forward.

WHAT DO you love about yourself or what are you learning to love?

_____

_____

_____

_____

_____

_____

_____

_____

_____

WHEEL OF LIFE

THE WHEEL OF LIFE is a great tool to help you improve your life balance. It helps you quickly and graphically identify and gather information on the areas in your life to which you want to devote more energy, and helps you understand where you might want to intentionally cut back.

Start at the tip of the pie piece and color out to where you believe represents your current level of mastery in each of the areas.

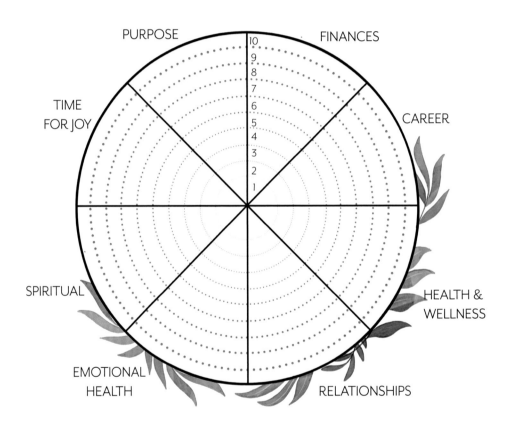

WHAT I'M proud of this month:

_____

_____

_____

_____

_____

INTENTIONS

INTENTION 1: _____

_____

_____

_____

_____

INTENTION 2: _____

_____

_____

_____

_____

INTENTION 3: _____

_____

_____

_____

_____

INTENTION 4: _____

_____

_____

_____

_____

INTENTION 5: _____

_____

_____

_____

_____

EMOTIONAL VIBRATION CHART

CONTEMPLATE THE emotions you've been feeling recently. On the chart, circle the emotions that most closely depict how you've felt over the past month or so.

ENLIGHTENMENT

PEACE

JOY

LOVE

REASON

ACCEPTANCE

WILLINGNESS

NEUTRALITY

COURAGE

PRIDE

ANGER

DESIRE

FEAR

GRIEF

APATHY

GUILT

SHAME

NOTES:

_____

_____

_____

_____

_____

_____

_____

_____

_____

_____

_____

_____

_____

_____

_____

_____

_____

_____

NURTURE TRACKER

NURTURE

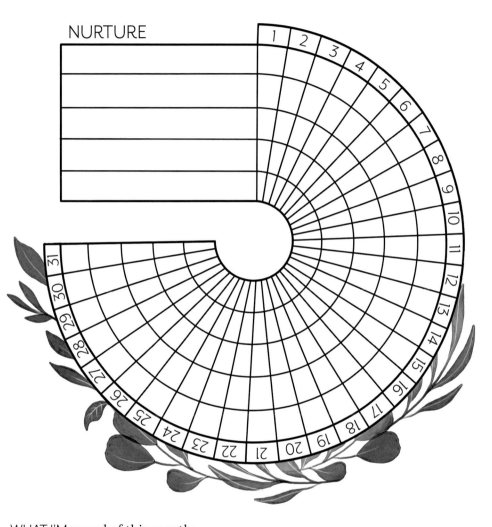

WHAT I'M proud of this month:

_____
_____
_____
_____
_____
_____
_____

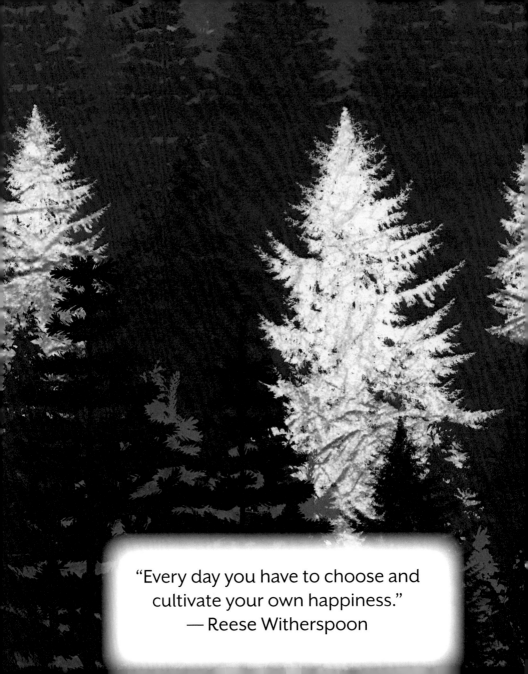

"Every day you have to choose and cultivate your own happiness."
— Reese Witherspoon

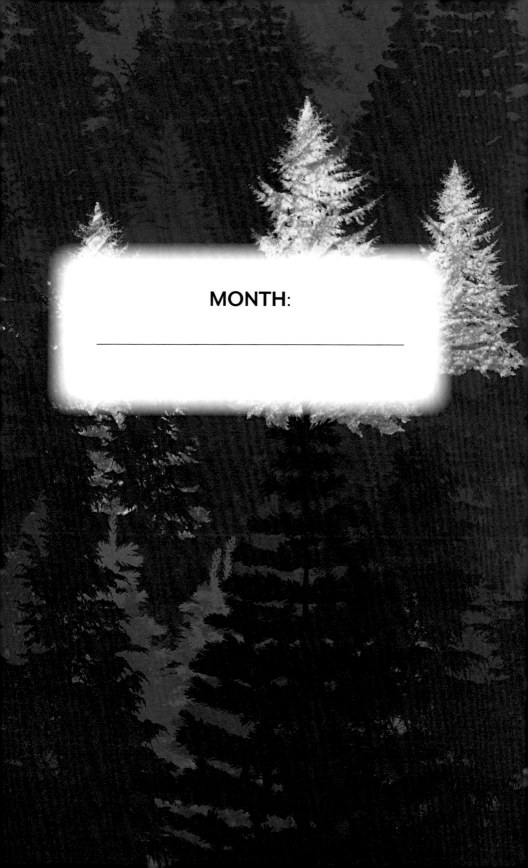

MONTH:

_____

WHAT IS the situation or circumstances that put you in the face of adversity, a traumatic time or difficult experience? This may include —but is not limited to physical injury, illness, loss, financial issues, mental strain or emotional harm. What's your story?

_____

_____

_____

_____

_____

_____

_____

_____

_____

_____

_____

_____

_____

_____

_____

_____

_____

_____

_____

_____

_____

_____

_____

_____

USE THIS space to capture additional details about where you were, what you were doing and how this impacted your life. What other contributing factors or people were involved?

_____

_____

_____

_____

_____

_____

_____

_____

_____

_____

_____

_____

WHAT WAS your mindset at the time? Use this area to jot down the feelings you processed. Did you feel fear, anger, frustration, overwhelm, devastation, disbelief or optimism? What feelings are coming up for you now about your story?

_____

_____

_____

_____

_____

_____

_____

_____

_____

_____

_____

_____

_____

_____

WHAT DID you do next? Think back to that time and try to recall what you did next. What, if anything, would you do differently?

_____

_____

_____

_____

_____

_____

_____

_____

_____

_____

_____

_____

_____

WHAT WAS—or is—holding you back from moving forward on your path?

_____

_____

_____

_____

_____

_____

_____

_____

_____

_____

_____

_____

_____

_____

BREATHE

WHEN YOU find yourself stuck, stressed or emotionally heightened, you can try a technique called box breathing to gather and recenter yourself. It's a simple practice and easy to learn. It can help you increase your concentration, bring you back to the moment and feel grounded so you can continue moving forward on your path. You can do this anywhere at any time. Box breathing can be done lying down or seated.

FOUR BASIC STEPS FOR BOX BREATHING, EACH LASTING FOUR SECONDS:

1. Breathe in slowly for a count of four. Feel the air fill your lungs.

2. Hold your breath for a count of four, trying not to inhale or exhale.

3. Slowly release your breath, exhaling through your mouth for four seconds.

4. Hold your breath for another four-count.

Repeat these steps until you feel as though you've gathered yourself.

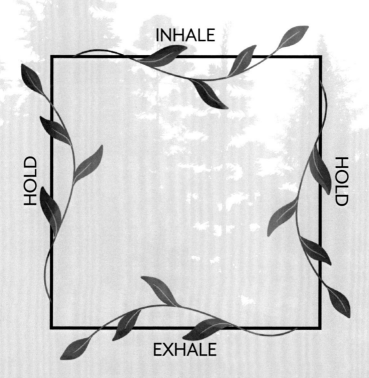

RESEARCH AND make a list of resources that can help you gain a better understanding of what information you'd like to gather. Ideas for your list could include books, personal development courses, workshops, retreats, conferences, websites, blogs, newsletters, mentorship, articles, videos, podcasts, apps and more. Be sure to connect with me on Instagram (@ginnypriem) where I'll share a variety of resources.

-
-
-
-
-
-
-
-
-

KEY LEARNINGS FROM RESOURCES:

_____
_____
_____
_____
_____
_____
_____
_____
_____

WHAT HAVE you discovered about yourself and your situation?

_____

_____

_____

_____

_____

_____

_____

_____

_____

WHAT ELSE would you like to gather and understand?

_____

_____

_____

_____

_____

_____

_____

_____

_____

_____

WHAT'S NEXT on your path? Where would you like to go from here?

_____

_____

_____

_____

_____

_____

_____

_____

_____

_____

DO YOU engage in negative self-talk or hold a self-limiting belief you tell yourself or have told yourself in the past? If you're able, close your eyes and say this to yourself one time.

JOURNAL PROMPT: What did that bring up for you when you spoke to yourself in a negative way?

_____

_____

_____

_____

_____

_____

_____

_____

_____

Take that negative self-talk and flip the script. Try saying the opposite. If that doesn't feel possible right now, try something 10% kinder. Close your eyes again and say this kinder thought to yourself three times, maybe even with a smile on your face.

JOURNAL PROMPT: How do you feel speaking in a more kind, positive way to yourself?

_____

_____

_____

_____

_____

_____

_____

THINK ABOUT how your intentions or self-limiting thoughts have potentially been shaping your feelings and contributing to your overall happiness. What would you like to be intentional about that can bring you more peace and joy in your life?

_____

_____

_____

_____

_____

_____

_____

_____

_____

_____

_____

What you believe, you can become.
You're not defined by what happened to you,
but you can define your path forward.

WHAT DO you love about yourself or what are you learning to love?

_____

_____

_____

_____

_____

_____

_____

_____

_____

_____

WHEEL OF LIFE

THE WHEEL OF LIFE is a great tool to help you improve your life balance. It helps you quickly and graphically identify and gather information on the areas in your life to which you want to devote more energy, and helps you understand where you might want to intentionally cut back.

Start at the tip of the pie piece and color out to where you believe represents your current level of mastery in each of the areas.

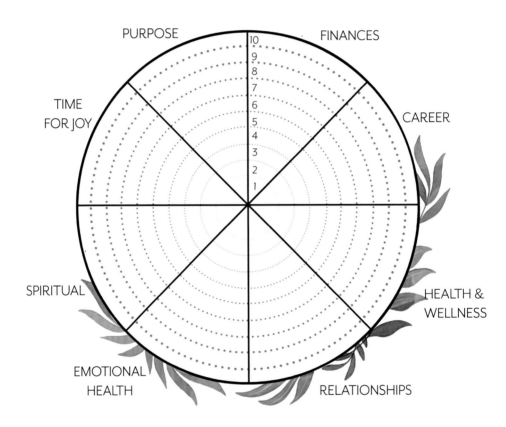

WHAT I'M proud of this month:

_____

_____

_____

_____

_____

INTENTIONS

INTENTION 1: _____
_____
_____
_____
_____

INTENTION 2: _____
_____
_____
_____
_____

INTENTION 3: _____
_____
_____
_____
_____

INTENTION 4: _____
_____
_____
_____
_____

INTENTION 5: _____
_____
_____
_____
_____

EMOTIONAL VIBRATION CHART

CONTEMPLATE THE emotions you've been feeling recently. On the chart, circle the emotions that most closely depict how you've felt over the past month or so.

ENLIGHTENMENT

PEACE

JOY

LOVE

REASON

ACCEPTANCE

WILLINGNESS

NEUTRALITY

COURAGE

PRIDE

ANGER

DESIRE

FEAR

GRIEF

APATHY

GUILT

SHAME

NOTES:

_____
_____
_____
_____
_____
_____
_____
_____
_____
_____
_____
_____
_____
_____
_____
_____
_____
_____
_____
_____

NURTURE TRACKER

NURTURE

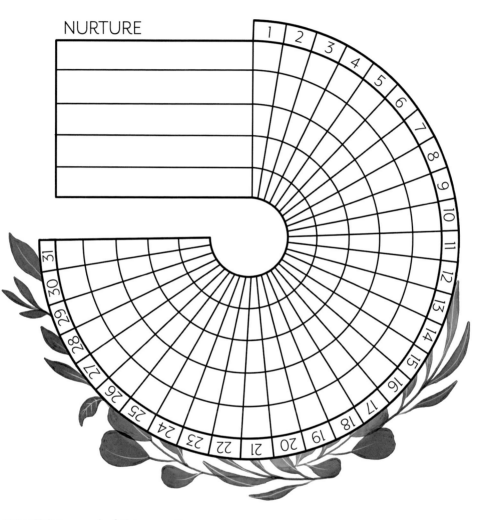

WHAT I'M proud of this month:

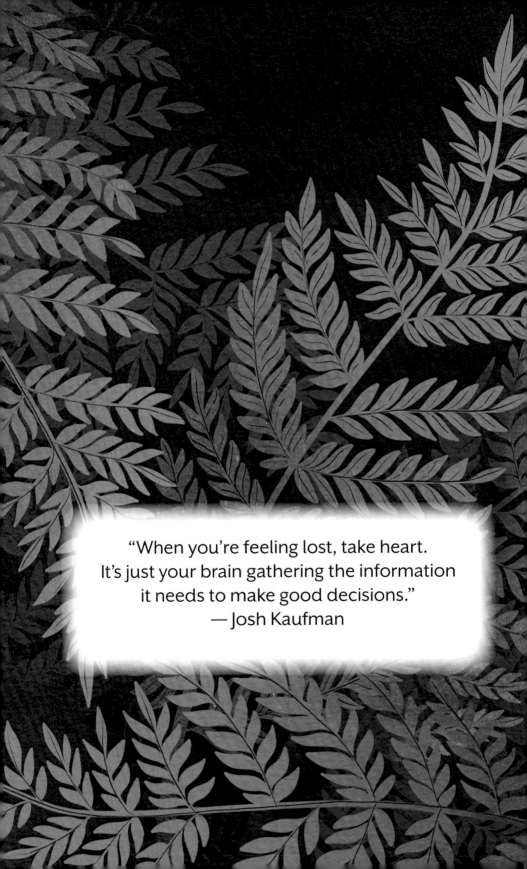

"When you're feeling lost, take heart.
It's just your brain gathering the information
it needs to make good decisions."
— Josh Kaufman

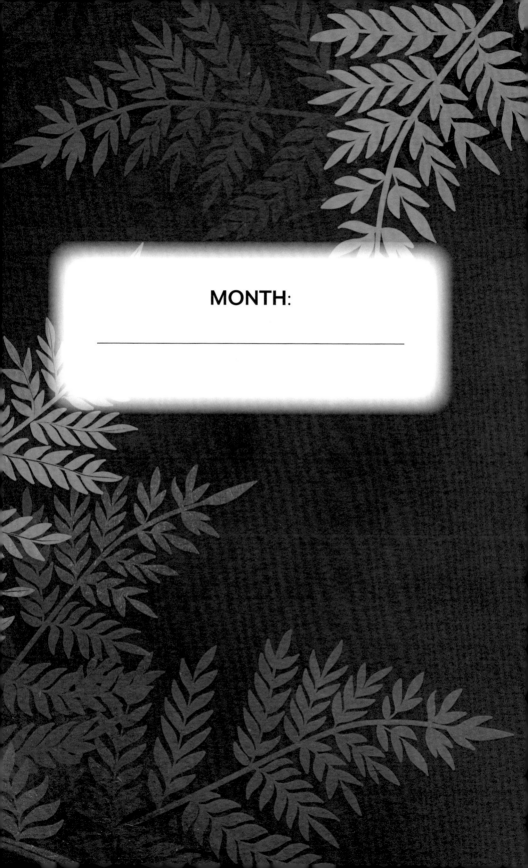

MONTH:

_____

WHAT IS the situation or circumstances that put you in the face of adversity, a traumatic time or difficult experience? This may include —but is not limited to physical injury, illness, loss, financial issues, mental strain or emotional harm. What's your story?

_____

_____

_____

_____

_____

_____

_____

_____

_____

_____

_____

_____

_____

_____

_____

_____

_____

_____

_____

_____

_____

_____

_____

_____

_____

_____

_____

USE THIS space to capture additional details about where you were, what you were doing and how this impacted your life. What other contributing factors or people were involved?

_____

_____

_____

_____

_____

_____

_____

_____

_____

_____

_____

WHAT WAS your mindset at the time? Use this area to jot down the feelings you processed. Did you feel fear, anger, frustration, overwhelm, devastation, disbelief or optimism? What feelings are coming up for you now about your story?

_____

_____

_____

_____

_____

_____

_____

_____

_____

_____

_____

_____

_____

WHAT DID you do next? Think back to that time and try to recall what you did next. What, if anything, would you do differently?

_____

_____

_____

_____

_____

_____

_____

_____

_____

_____

_____

_____

_____

WHAT WAS—or is—holding you back from moving forward on your path?

_____

_____

_____

_____

_____

_____

_____

_____

_____

_____

_____

_____

_____

_____

BREATHE

WHEN YOU find yourself stuck, stressed or emotionally heightened, you can try a technique called box breathing to gather and recenter yourself. It's a simple practice and easy to learn. It can help you increase your concentration, bring you back to the moment and feel grounded so you can continue moving forward on your path. You can do this anywhere at any time. Box breathing can be done lying down or seated.

FOUR BASIC STEPS FOR BOX BREATHING, EACH LASTING FOUR SECONDS:

1. Breathe in slowly for a count of four. Feel the air fill your lungs.

2. Hold your breath for a count of four, trying not to inhale or exhale.

3. Slowly release your breath, exhaling through your mouth for four seconds.

4. Hold your breath for another four-count.

Repeat these steps until you feel as though you've gathered yourself.

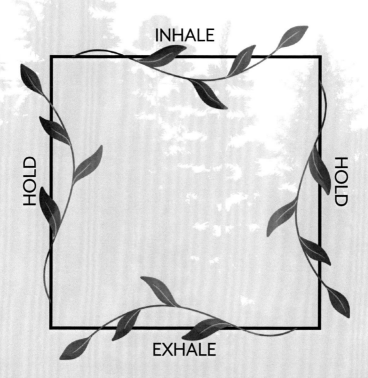

INHALE

HOLD

HOLD

EXHALE

RESEARCH AND make a list of resources that can help you gain a better understanding of what information you'd like to gather. Ideas for your list could include books, personal development courses, workshops, retreats, conferences, websites, blogs, newsletters, mentorship, articles, videos, podcasts, apps and more. Be sure to connect with me on Instagram (@ginnypriem) where I'll share a variety of resources.

-
-
-
-
-
-
-
-
-
-

KEY LEARNINGS FROM RESOURCES:

_____
_____
_____
_____
_____
_____
_____
_____

WHAT HAVE you discovered about yourself and your situation?

_____

_____

_____

_____

_____

_____

_____

_____

_____

WHAT ELSE would you like to gather and understand?

_____

_____

_____

_____

_____

_____

_____

_____

_____

WHAT'S NEXT on your path? Where would you like to go from here?

_____

_____

_____

_____

_____

_____

_____

_____

_____

DO YOU engage in negative self-talk or hold a self-limiting belief you tell yourself or have told yourself in the past? If you're able, close your eyes and say this to yourself one time.

JOURNAL PROMPT: What did that bring up for you when you spoke to yourself in a negative way?

_____

_____

_____

_____

_____

_____

_____

_____

_____

Take that negative self-talk and flip the script. Try saying the opposite. If that doesn't feel possible right now, try something 10% kinder. Close your eyes again and say this kinder thought to yourself three times, maybe even with a smile on your face.

JOURNAL PROMPT: How do you feel speaking in a more kind, positive way to yourself?

_____

_____

_____

_____

_____

_____

_____

THINK ABOUT how your intentions or self-limiting thoughts have potentially been shaping your feelings and contributing to your overall happiness. What would you like to be intentional about that can bring you more peace and joy in your life?

_____

_____

_____

_____

_____

_____

_____

_____

_____

_____

What you believe, you can become.
You're not defined by what happened to you,
but you can define your path forward.

WHAT DO you love about yourself or what are you learning to love?

_____

_____

_____

_____

_____

_____

_____

_____

_____

WHEEL OF LIFE

THE WHEEL OF LIFE is a great tool to help you improve your life balance. It helps you quickly and graphically identify and gather information on the areas in your life to which you want to devote more energy, and helps you understand where you might want to intentionally cut back.

Start at the tip of the pie piece and color out to where you believe represents your current level of mastery in each of the areas.

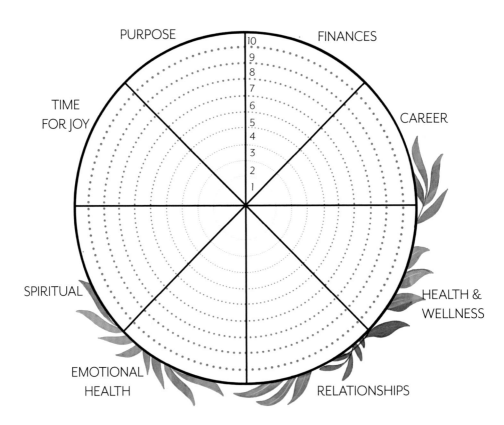

WHAT I'M proud of this month:

_____

_____

_____

_____

_____

INTENTIONS

INTENTION 1: _____
_____
_____
_____
_____

INTENTION 2: _____
_____
_____
_____
_____

INTENTION 3: _____
_____
_____
_____
_____

INTENTION 4: _____
_____
_____
_____
_____

INTENTION 5: _____
_____
_____
_____
_____

EMOTIONAL VIBRATION CHART

CONTEMPLATE THE emotions you've been feeling recently. On the chart, circle the emotions that most closely depict how you've felt over the past month or so.

ENLIGHTENMENT

PEACE

JOY

LOVE

REASON

ACCEPTANCE

WILLINGNESS

NEUTRALITY

COURAGE

PRIDE

ANGER

DESIRE

FEAR

GRIEF

APATHY

GUILT

SHAME

NOTES:

_____

_____

_____

_____

_____

_____

_____

_____

_____

_____

_____

_____

_____

_____

_____

_____

_____

_____

NURTURE TRACKER

NURTURE

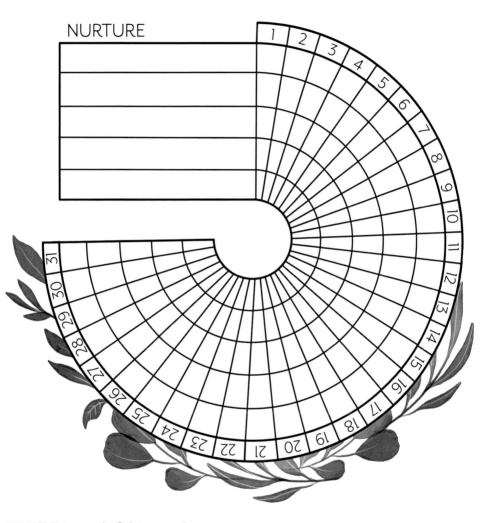

WHAT I'M proud of this month:

_____
_____
_____
_____
_____
_____
_____

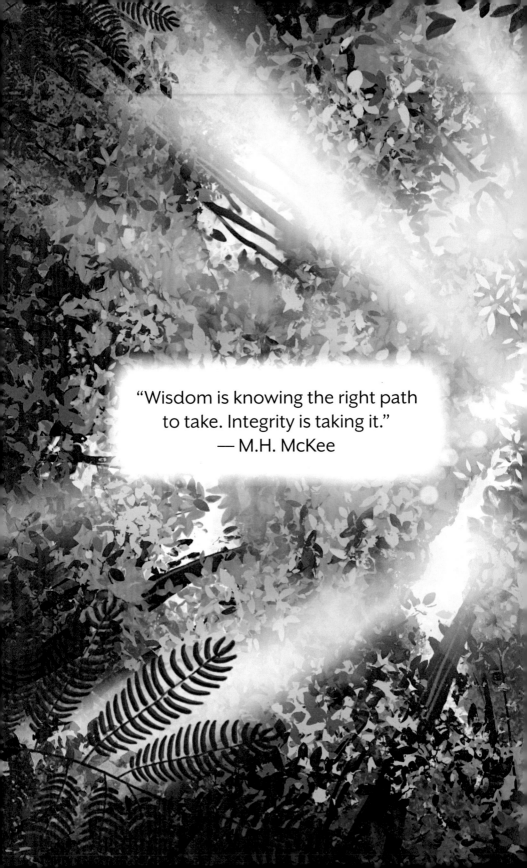

"Wisdom is knowing the right path
to take. Integrity is taking it."
— M.H. McKee

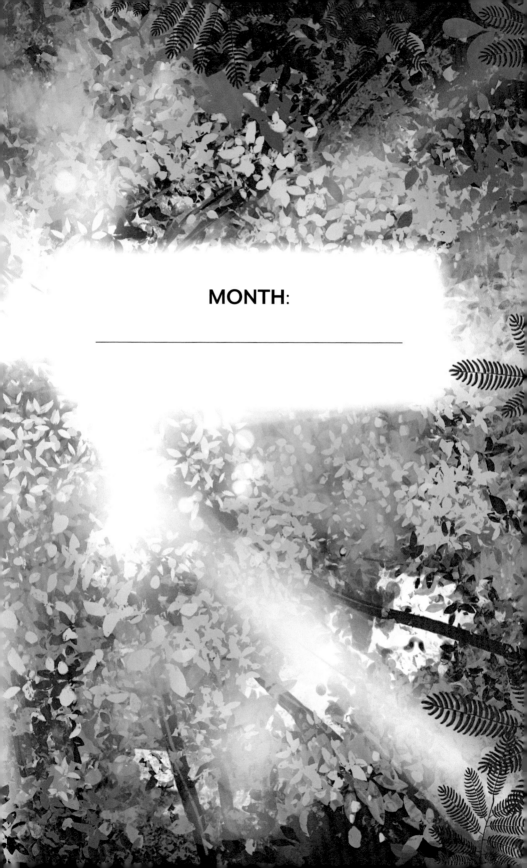

MONTH:

_____

WHAT IS the situation or circumstances that put you in the face of adversity, a traumatic time or difficult experience? This may include —but is not limited to— physical injury, illness, loss, financial issues, mental strain or emotional harm. What's your story?

_____

_____

_____

_____

_____

_____

_____

_____

_____

_____

_____

_____

_____

_____

_____

_____

_____

_____

_____

_____

_____

_____

_____

_____

_____

_____

_____

USE THIS space to capture additional details about where you were, what you were doing and how this impacted your life. What other contributing factors or people were involved?

_____
_____
_____
_____
_____
_____
_____
_____
_____
_____
_____

WHAT WAS your mindset at the time? Use this area to jot down the feelings you processed. Did you feel fear, anger, frustration, overwhelm, devastation, disbelief or optimism? What feelings are coming up for you now about your story?

_____
_____
_____
_____
_____
_____
_____
_____
_____
_____
_____
_____
_____

WHAT DID you do next? Think back to that time and try to recall what you did next. What, if anything, would you do differently?

_____

_____

_____

_____

_____

_____

_____

_____

_____

_____

_____

_____

_____

WHAT WAS—or is—holding you back from moving forward on your path?

_____

_____

_____

_____

_____

_____

_____

_____

_____

_____

_____

_____

_____

_____

BREATHE

WHEN YOU find yourself stuck, stressed or emotionally heightened, you can try a technique called box breathing to gather and recenter yourself. It's a simple practice and easy to learn. It can help you increase your concentration, bring you back to the moment and feel grounded so you can continue moving forward on your path. You can do this anywhere at any time. Box breathing can be done lying down or seated.

FOUR BASIC STEPS FOR BOX BREATHING, EACH LASTING FOUR SECONDS:

1. Breathe in slowly for a count of four. Feel the air fill your lungs.

2. Hold your breath for a count of four, trying not to inhale or exhale.

3. Slowly release your breath, exhaling through your mouth for four seconds.

4. Hold your breath for another four-count.

Repeat these steps until you feel as though you've gathered yourself.

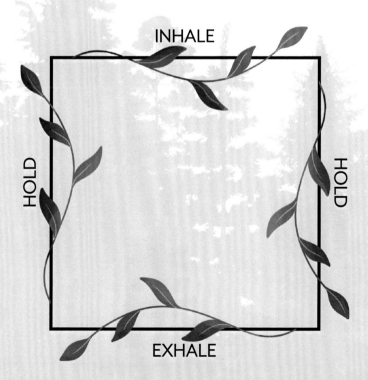

RESEARCH AND make a list of resources that can help you gain a better understanding of what information you'd like to gather. Ideas for your list could include books, personal development courses, workshops, retreats, conferences, websites, blogs, newsletters, mentorship, articles, videos, podcasts, apps and more. Be sure to connect with me on Instagram (@ginnypriem) where I'll share a variety of resources.

-
-
-
-
-
-
-
-
-

KEY LEARNINGS FROM RESOURCES:

_____
_____
_____
_____
_____
_____
_____
_____

WHAT HAVE you discovered about yourself and your situation?

_____

_____

_____

_____

_____

_____

_____

_____

_____

WHAT ELSE would you like to gather and understand?

_____

_____

_____

_____

_____

_____

_____

_____

WHAT'S NEXT on your path? Where would you like to go from here?

_____

_____

_____

_____

_____

_____

_____

_____

_____

DO YOU engage in negative self-talk or hold a self-limiting belief you tell yourself or have told yourself in the past? If you're able, close your eyes and say this to yourself one time.

JOURNAL PROMPT: What did that bring up for you when you spoke to yourself in a negative way?

_____

_____

_____

_____

_____

_____

_____

_____

_____

Take that negative self-talk and flip the script. Try saying the opposite. If that doesn't feel possible right now, try something 10% kinder. Close your eyes again and say this kinder thought to yourself three times, maybe even with a smile on your face.

JOURNAL PROMPT: How do you feel speaking in a more kind, positive way to yourself?

_____

_____

_____

_____

_____

_____

_____

THINK ABOUT how your intentions or self-limiting thoughts have potentially been shaping your feelings and contributing to your overall happiness. What would you like to be intentional about that can bring you more peace and joy in your life?

_____
_____
_____
_____
_____
_____
_____
_____
_____
_____

What you believe, you can become.
You're not defined by what happened to you,
but you can define your path forward.

WHAT DO you love about yourself or what are you learning to love?

_____
_____
_____
_____
_____
_____
_____
_____
_____
_____

WHEEL OF LIFE

THE WHEEL OF LIFE is a great tool to help you improve your life balance. It helps you quickly and graphically identify and gather information on the areas in your life to which you want to devote more energy, and helps you understand where you might want to intentionally cut back.

Start at the tip of the pie piece and color out to where you believe represents your current level of mastery in each of the areas.

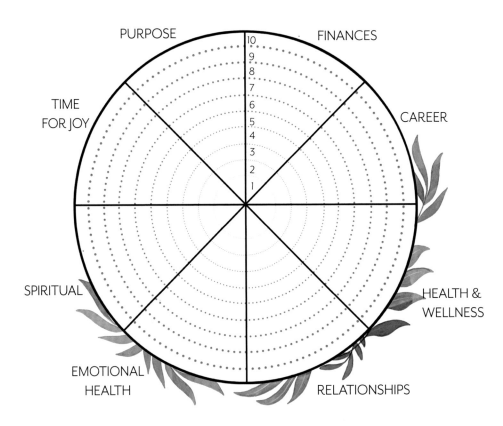

WHAT I'M proud of this month:

_____
_____
_____
_____
_____

INTENTIONS

INTENTION 1: _____
_____
_____
_____
_____

INTENTION 2: _____
_____
_____
_____
_____

INTENTION 3: _____
_____
_____
_____
_____

INTENTION 4: _____
_____
_____
_____
_____

INTENTION 5: _____
_____
_____
_____
_____

EMOTIONAL VIBRATION CHART

CONTEMPLATE THE emotions you've been feeling recently. On the chart, circle the emotions that most closely depict how you've felt over the past month or so.

ENLIGHTENMENT

PEACE

JOY

LOVE

REASON

ACCEPTANCE

WILLINGNESS

NEUTRALITY

COURAGE

PRIDE

ANGER

DESIRE

FEAR

GRIEF

APATHY

GUILT

SHAME

NOTES:

_____

_____

_____

_____

_____

_____

_____

_____

_____

_____

_____

_____

_____

_____

_____

_____

_____

_____

_____

_____

NURTURE TRACKER

NURTURE

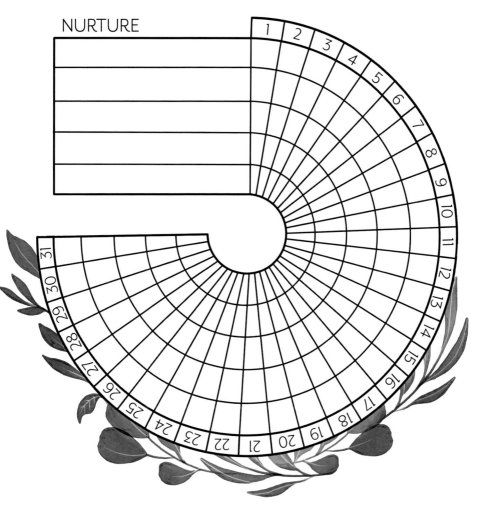

WHAT I'M proud of this month:

_____
_____
_____
_____
_____
_____
_____

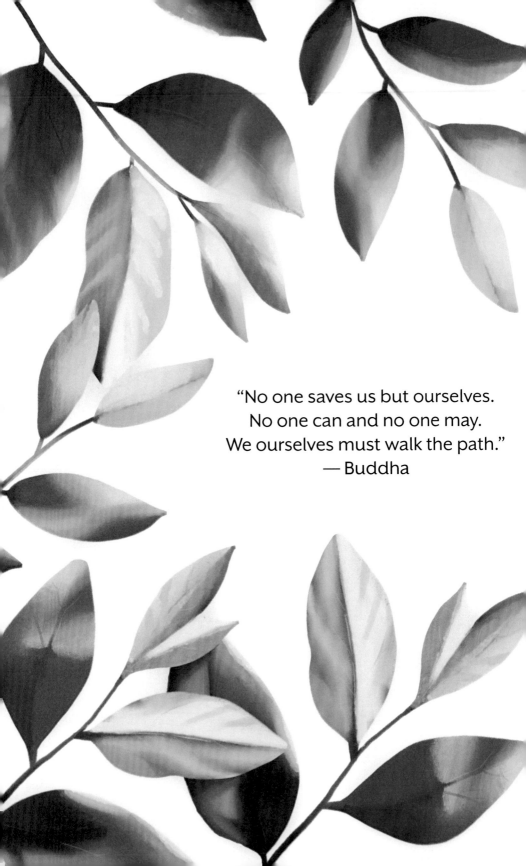

"No one saves us but ourselves.
No one can and no one may.
We ourselves must walk the path."
— Buddha

MONTH:

_____

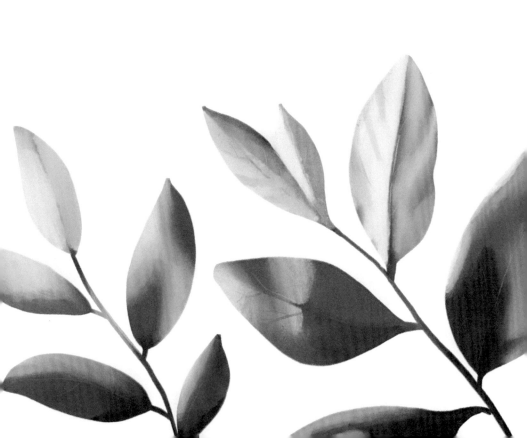

WHAT IS the situation or circumstances that put you in the face of adversity, a traumatic time or difficult experience? This may include —but is not limited to— physical injury, illness, loss, financial issues, mental strain or emotional harm. What's your story?

USE THIS space to capture additional details about where you were, what you were doing and how this impacted your life. What other contributing factors or people were involved?

_____

_____

_____

_____

_____

_____

_____

_____

_____

_____

_____

WHAT WAS your mindset at the time? Use this area to jot down the feelings you processed. Did you feel fear, anger, frustration, overwhelm, devastation, disbelief or optimism? What feelings are coming up for you now about your story?

_____

_____

_____

_____

_____

_____

_____

_____

_____

_____

_____

_____

_____

WHAT DID you do next? Think back to that time and try to recall what you did next. What, if anything, would you do differently?

_____

_____

_____

_____

_____

_____

_____

_____

_____

_____

_____

_____

_____

_____

WHAT WAS—or is—holding you back from moving forward on your path?

_____

_____

_____

_____

_____

_____

_____

_____

_____

_____

_____

_____

_____

BREATHE

WHEN YOU find yourself stuck, stressed or emotionally heightened, you can try a technique called box breathing to gather and recenter yourself. It's a simple practice and easy to learn. It can help you increase your concentration, bring you back to the moment and feel grounded so you can continue moving forward on your path. You can do this anywhere at any time. Box breathing can be done lying down or seated.

FOUR BASIC STEPS FOR BOX BREATHING, EACH LASTING FOUR SECONDS:

1. Breathe in slowly for a count of four. Feel the air fill your lungs.

2. Hold your breath for a count of four, trying not to inhale or exhale.

3. Slowly release your breath, exhaling through your mouth for four seconds.

4. Hold your breath for another four-count.

Repeat these steps until you feel as though you've gathered yourself.

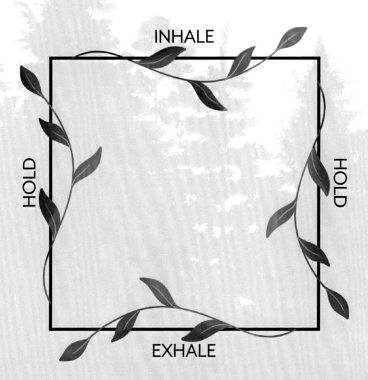

INHALE

HOLD

HOLD

EXHALE

RESEARCH AND make a list of resources that can help you gain a better understanding of what information you'd like to gather. Ideas for your list could include books, personal development courses, workshops, retreats, conferences, websites, blogs, newsletters, mentorship, articles, videos, podcasts, apps and more. Be sure to connect with me on Instagram (@ginnypriem) where I'll share a variety of resources.

-
-
-
-
-
-
-
-
-

KEY LEARNINGS FROM RESOURCES:

_____
_____
_____
_____
_____
_____
_____
_____

WHAT HAVE you discovered about yourself and your situation?

_____

_____

_____

_____

_____

_____

_____

_____

_____

WHAT ELSE would you like to gather and understand?

_____

_____

_____

_____

_____

_____

_____

_____

WHAT'S NEXT on your path? Where would you like to go from here?

_____

_____

_____

_____

_____

_____

_____

_____

_____

_____

DO YOU engage in negative self-talk or hold a self-limiting belief you tell yourself or have told yourself in the past? If you're able, close your eyes and say this to yourself one time.

JOURNAL PROMPT: What did that bring up for you when you spoke to yourself in a negative way?

_____

_____

_____

_____

_____

_____

_____

_____

_____

Take that negative self-talk and flip the script. Try saying the opposite. If that doesn't feel possible right now, try something 10% kinder. Close your eyes again and say this kinder thought to yourself three times, maybe even with a smile on your face.

JOURNAL PROMPT: How do you feel speaking in a more kind, positive way to yourself?

_____

_____

_____

_____

_____

_____

_____

THINK ABOUT how your intentions or self-limiting thoughts have potentially been shaping your feelings and contributing to your overall happiness. What would you like to be intentional about that can bring you more peace and joy in your life?

_____

_____

_____

_____

_____

_____

_____

_____

_____

_____

_____

What you believe, you can become.
You're not defined by what happened to you,
but you can define your path forward.

WHAT DO you love about yourself or what are you learning to love?

_____

_____

_____

_____

_____

_____

_____

_____

_____

_____

WHEEL OF LIFE

THE WHEEL OF LIFE is a great tool to help you improve your life balance. It helps you quickly and graphically identify and gather information on the areas in your life to which you want to devote more energy, and helps you understand where you might want to intentionally cut back.

Start at the tip of the pie piece and color out to where you believe represents your current level of mastery in each of the areas.

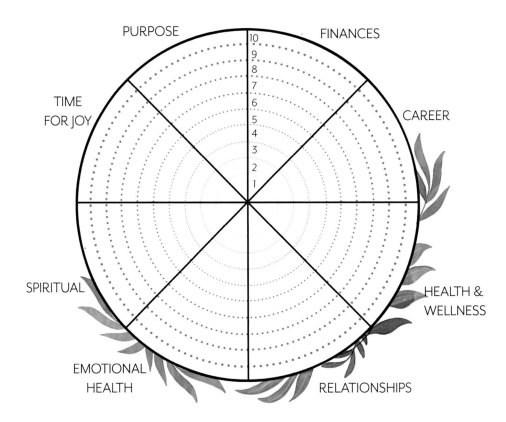

WHAT I'M proud of this month:

_____

_____

_____

_____

_____

INTENTIONS

INTENTION 1: _____
_____
_____
_____
_____

INTENTION 2: _____
_____
_____
_____
_____

INTENTION 3: _____
_____
_____
_____
_____

INTENTION 4: _____
_____
_____
_____
_____

INTENTION 5: _____
_____
_____
_____
_____

EMOTIONAL VIBRATION CHART

CONTEMPLATE THE emotions you've been feeling recently. On the chart, circle the emotions that most closely depict how you've felt over the past month or so.

ENLIGHTENMENT

PEACE

JOY

LOVE

REASON

ACCEPTANCE

WILLINGNESS

NEUTRALITY

COURAGE

PRIDE

ANGER

DESIRE

FEAR

GRIEF

APATHY

GUILT

SHAME

NOTES:

_____
_____
_____
_____
_____
_____
_____
_____
_____
_____
_____
_____
_____
_____
_____
_____
_____
_____
_____
_____

NURTURE TRACKER

NURTURE

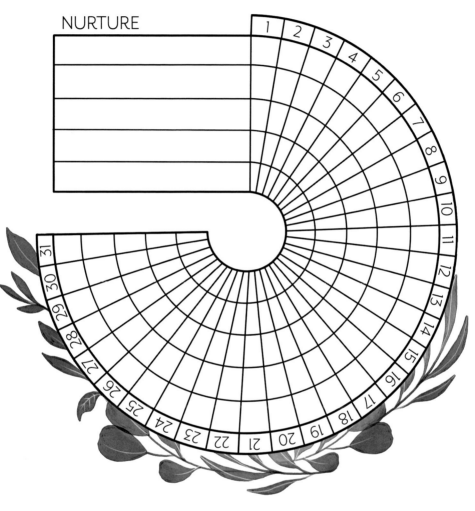

WHAT I'M proud of this month:

_____
_____
_____
_____
_____
_____
_____

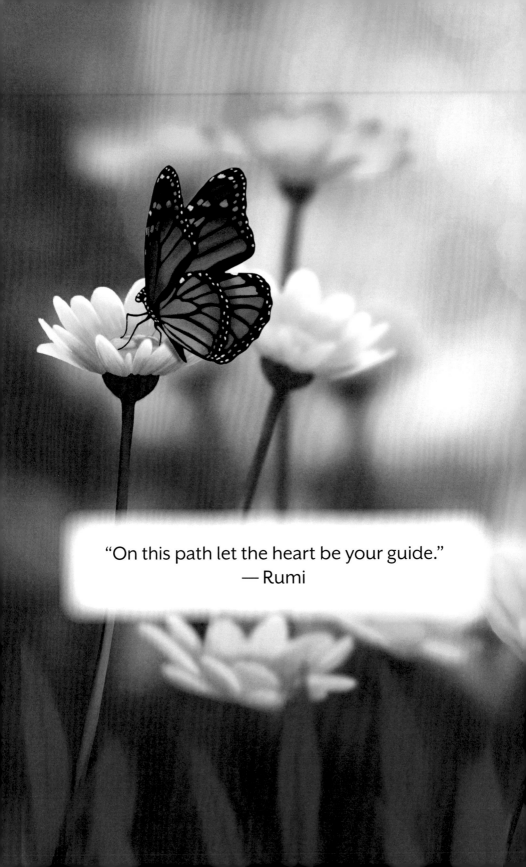

"On this path let the heart be your guide."
— Rumi

MONTH:

_____

WHAT IS the situation or circumstances that put you in the face of adversity, a traumatic time or difficult experience? This may include —but is not limited to— physical injury, illness, loss, financial issues, mental strain or emotional harm. What's your story?

_____

_____

_____

_____

_____

_____

_____

_____

_____

_____

_____

_____

_____

_____

_____

_____

_____

_____

_____

_____

_____

_____

_____

_____

_____

USE THIS space to capture additional details about where you were, what you were doing and how this impacted your life. What other contributing factors or people were involved?

_____

_____

_____

_____

_____

_____

_____

_____

_____

_____

_____

_____

WHAT WAS your mindset at the time? Use this area to jot down the feelings you processed. Did you feel fear, anger, frustration, overwhelm, devastation, disbelief or optimism? What feelings are coming up for you now about your story?

_____

_____

_____

_____

_____

_____

_____

_____

_____

_____

_____

_____

_____

_____

WHAT DID you do next? Think back to that time and try to recall what you did next. What, if anything, would you do differently?

_____

_____

_____

_____

_____

_____

_____

_____

_____

_____

_____

_____

_____

_____

WHAT WAS—or is—holding you back from moving forward on your path?

_____

_____

_____

_____

_____

_____

_____

_____

_____

_____

_____

_____

_____

_____

BREATHE

WHEN YOU find yourself stuck, stressed or emotionally heightened, you can try a technique called box breathing to gather and recenter yourself. It's a simple practice and easy to learn. It can help you increase your concentration, bring you back to the moment and feel grounded so you can continue moving forward on your path. You can do this anywhere at any time. Box breathing can be done lying down or seated.

FOUR BASIC STEPS FOR BOX BREATHING, EACH LASTING FOUR SECONDS:

1. Breathe in slowly for a count of four. Feel the air fill your lungs.

2. Hold your breath for a count of four, trying not to inhale or exhale.

3. Slowly release your breath, exhaling through your mouth for four seconds.

4. Hold your breath for another four-count.

Repeat these steps until you feel as though you've gathered yourself.

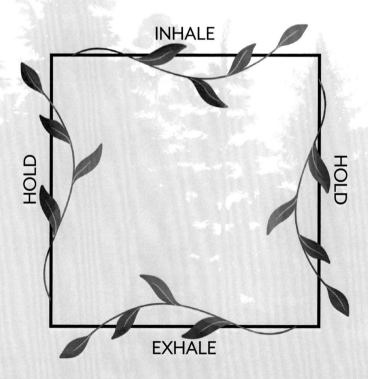

RESEARCH AND make a list of resources that can help you gain a better understanding of what information you'd like to gather. Ideas for your list could include books, personal development courses, workshops, retreats, conferences, websites, blogs, newsletters, mentorship, articles, videos, podcasts, apps and more. Be sure to connect with me on Instagram (@ginnypriem) where I'll share a variety of resources.

-
-
-
-
-
-
-
-
-
-

KEY LEARNINGS FROM RESOURCES:

_____
_____
_____
_____
_____
_____
_____
_____

WHAT HAVE you discovered about yourself and your situation?

_____
_____
_____
_____
_____
_____
_____
_____
_____

WHAT ELSE would you like to gather and understand?

_____
_____
_____
_____
_____
_____
_____
_____

WHAT'S NEXT on your path? Where would you like to go from here?

_____
_____
_____
_____
_____
_____
_____
_____
_____

DO YOU engage in negative self-talk or hold a self-limiting belief you tell yourself or have told yourself in the past? If you're able, close your eyes and say this to yourself one time.

JOURNAL PROMPT: What did that bring up for you when you spoke to yourself in a negative way?

_____

_____

_____

_____

_____

_____

_____

_____

Take that negative self-talk and flip the script. Try saying the opposite. If that doesn't feel possible right now, try something 10% kinder. Close your eyes again and say this kinder thought to yourself three times, maybe even with a smile on your face.

JOURNAL PROMPT: How do you feel speaking in a more kind, positive way to yourself?

_____

_____

_____

_____

_____

_____

_____

THINK ABOUT how your intentions or self-limiting thoughts have potentially been shaping your feelings and contributing to your overall happiness. What would you like to be intentional about that can bring you more peace and joy in your life?

_____

_____

_____

_____

_____

_____

_____

_____

_____

_____

_____

What you believe, you can become.
You're not defined by what happened to you,
but you can define your path forward.

WHAT DO you love about yourself or what are you learning to love?

_____

_____

_____

_____

_____

_____

_____

_____

_____

_____

WHEEL OF LIFE

THE WHEEL OF LIFE is a great tool to help you improve your life balance. It helps you quickly and graphically identify and gather information on the areas in your life to which you want to devote more energy, and helps you understand where you might want to intentionally cut back.

Start at the tip of the pie piece and color out to where you believe represents your current level of mastery in each of the areas.

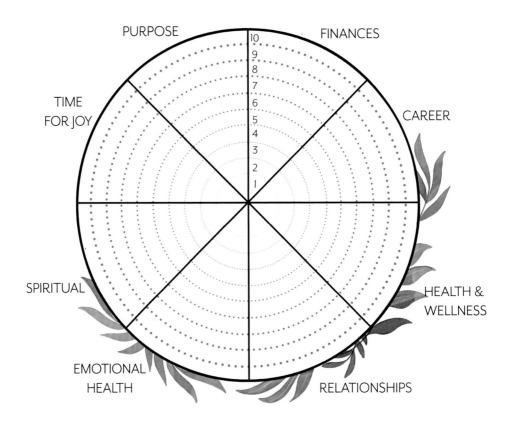

WHAT I'M proud of this month:

_____

_____

_____

_____

_____

INTENTIONS

INTENTION 1: _____

_____

_____

_____

_____

INTENTION 2: _____

_____

_____

_____

_____

INTENTION 3: _____

_____

_____

_____

_____

INTENTION 4: _____

_____

_____

_____

_____

INTENTION 5: _____

_____

_____

_____

_____

EMOTIONAL VIBRATION CHART

CONTEMPLATE THE emotions you've been feeling recently. On the chart, circle the emotions that most closely depict how you've felt over the past month or so.

ENLIGHTENMENT

PEACE

JOY

LOVE

REASON

ACCEPTANCE

WILLINGNESS

NEUTRALITY

COURAGE

PRIDE

ANGER

DESIRE

FEAR

GRIEF

APATHY

GUILT

SHAME

NOTES:

_____

_____

_____

_____

_____

_____

_____

_____

_____

_____

_____

_____

_____

_____

_____

_____

_____

_____

NURTURE TRACKER

NURTURE

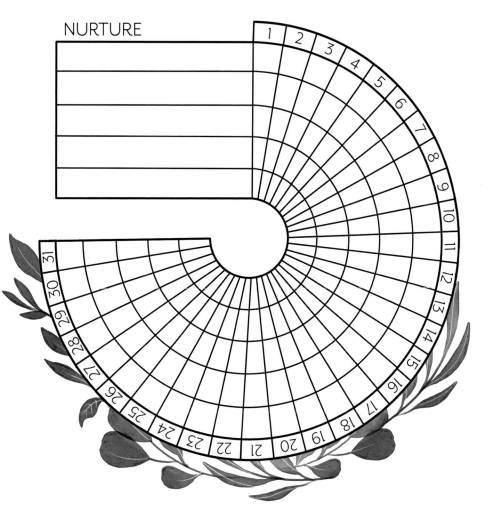

WHAT I'M proud of this month:

_____
_____
_____
_____
_____
_____
_____

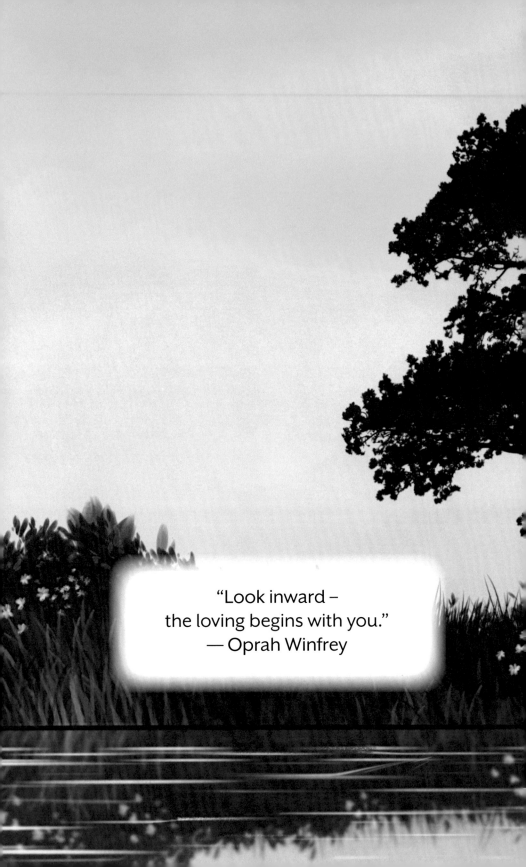

"Look inward –
the loving begins with you."
— Oprah Winfrey

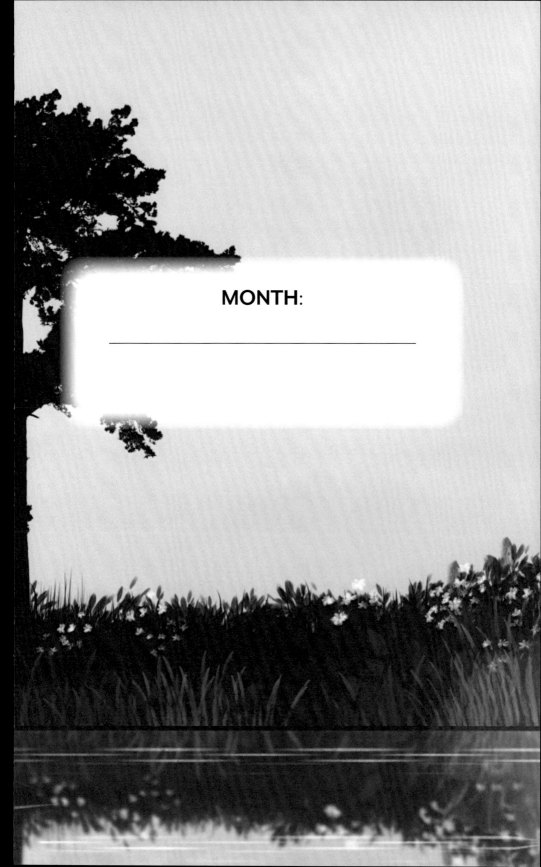

MONTH:
_____

WHAT IS the situation or circumstances that put you in the face of adversity, a traumatic time or difficult experience? This may include —but is not limited to— physical injury, illness, loss, financial issues, mental strain or emotional harm. What's your story?

_____

_____

_____

_____

_____

_____

_____

_____

_____

_____

_____

_____

_____

_____

_____

_____

_____

_____

_____

_____

_____

_____

_____

_____

USE THIS space to capture additional details about where you were, what you were doing and how this impacted your life. What other contributing factors or people were involved?

_____

_____

_____

_____

_____

_____

_____

_____

_____

_____

_____

WHAT WAS your mindset at the time? Use this area to jot down the feelings you processed. Did you feel fear, anger, frustration, overwhelm, devastation, disbelief or optimism? What feelings are coming up for you now about your story?

_____

_____

_____

_____

_____

_____

_____

_____

_____

_____

_____

_____

_____

_____

WHAT DID you do next? Think back to that time and try to recall what you did next. What, if anything, would you do differently?

_____

_____

_____

_____

_____

_____

_____

_____

_____

_____

_____

_____

WHAT WAS—or is—holding you back from moving forward on your path?

_____

_____

_____

_____

_____

_____

_____

_____

_____

_____

_____

_____

_____

BREATHE

WHEN YOU find yourself stuck, stressed or emotionally heightened, you can try a technique called box breathing to gather and recenter yourself. It's a simple practice and easy to learn. It can help you increase your concentration, bring you back to the moment and feel grounded so you can continue moving forward on your path. You can do this anywhere at any time. Box breathing can be done lying down or seated.

FOUR BASIC STEPS FOR BOX BREATHING, EACH LASTING FOUR SECONDS:

1. Breathe in slowly for a count of four. Feel the air fill your lungs.

2. Hold your breath for a count of four, trying not to inhale or exhale.

3. Slowly release your breath, exhaling through your mouth for four seconds.

4. Hold your breath for another four-count.

Repeat these steps until you feel as though you've gathered yourself.

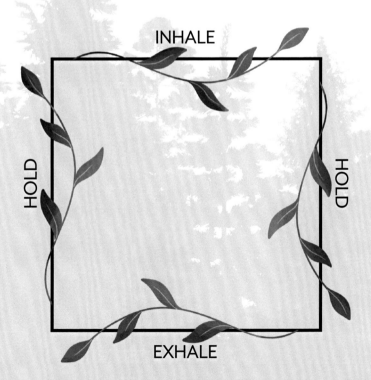

INHALE

HOLD

HOLD

EXHALE

RESEARCH AND make a list of resources that can help you gain a better understanding of what information you'd like to gather. Ideas for your list could include books, personal development courses, workshops, retreats, conferences, websites, blogs, newsletters, mentorship, articles, videos, podcasts, apps and more. Be sure to connect with me on Instagram (@ginnypriem) where I'll share a variety of resources.

-
-
-
-
-
-
-
-
-

KEY LEARNINGS FROM RESOURCES:

_____
_____
_____
_____
_____
_____
_____
_____
_____

WHAT HAVE you discovered about yourself and your situation?

_____

_____

_____

_____

_____

_____

_____

_____

_____

WHAT ELSE would you like to gather and understand?

_____

_____

_____

_____

_____

_____

_____

_____

_____

WHAT'S NEXT on your path? Where would you like to go from here?

_____

_____

_____

_____

_____

_____

_____

_____

_____

_____

DO YOU engage in negative self-talk or hold a self-limiting belief you tell yourself or have told yourself in the past? If you're able, close your eyes and say this to yourself one time.

JOURNAL PROMPT: What did that bring up for you when you spoke to yourself in a negative way?

_____

_____

_____

_____

_____

_____

_____

_____

_____

Take that negative self-talk and flip the script. Try saying the opposite.
If that doesn't feel possible right now, try something 10% kinder.
Close your eyes again and say this kinder thought to yourself
three times, maybe even with a smile on your face.

JOURNAL PROMPT: How do you feel speaking in a more kind, positive way to yourself?

_____

_____

_____

_____

_____

_____

_____

_____

THINK ABOUT how your intentions or self-limiting thoughts have potentially been shaping your feelings and contributing to your overall happiness. What would you like to be intentional about that can bring you more peace and joy in your life?

_____
_____
_____
_____
_____
_____
_____
_____
_____
_____
_____

What you believe, you can become.
You're not defined by what happened to you,
but you can define your path forward.

WHAT DO you love about yourself or what are you learning to love?

_____
_____
_____
_____
_____
_____
_____
_____
_____

WHEEL OF LIFE

THE WHEEL OF LIFE is a great tool to help you improve your life balance. It helps you quickly and graphically identify and gather information on the areas in your life to which you want to devote more energy, and helps you understand where you might want to intentionally cut back.

Start at the tip of the pie piece and color out to where you believe represents your current level of mastery in each of the areas.

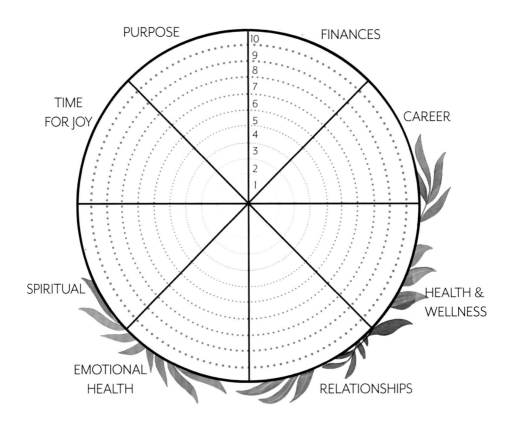

WHAT I'M proud of this month:

_____

_____

_____

_____

_____

INTENTIONS

INTENTION 1: _____
_____
_____
_____
_____

INTENTION 2: _____
_____
_____
_____
_____

INTENTION 3: _____
_____
_____
_____
_____

INTENTION 4: _____
_____
_____
_____
_____

INTENTION 5: _____
_____
_____
_____
_____

EMOTIONAL VIBRATION CHART

CONTEMPLATE THE emotions you've been feeling recently. On the chart, circle the emotions that most closely depict how you've felt over the past month or so.

ENLIGHTENMENT

PEACE

JOY

LOVE

REASON

ACCEPTANCE

WILLINGNESS

NEUTRALITY

COURAGE

PRIDE

ANGER

DESIRE

FEAR

GRIEF

APATHY

GUILT

SHAME

NOTES:

_____

_____

_____

_____

_____

_____

_____

_____

_____

_____

_____

_____

_____

_____

_____

_____

_____

_____

_____

_____

NURTURE TRACKER

NURTURE

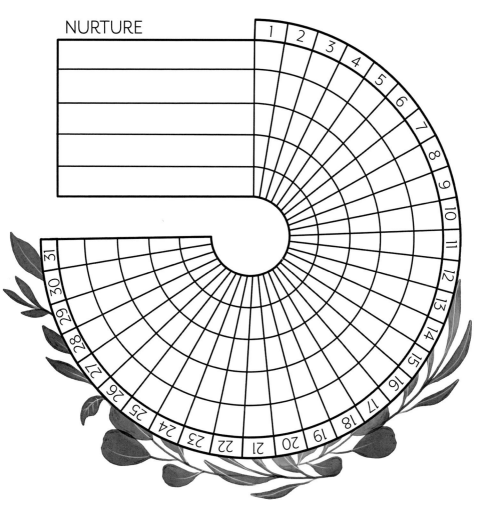

WHAT I'M proud of this month:

_____
_____
_____
_____
_____
_____
_____

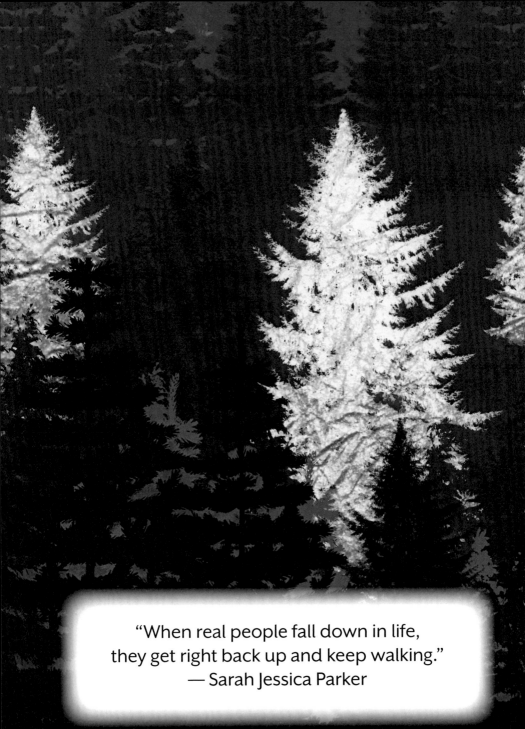

"When real people fall down in life,
they get right back up and keep walking."
— Sarah Jessica Parker

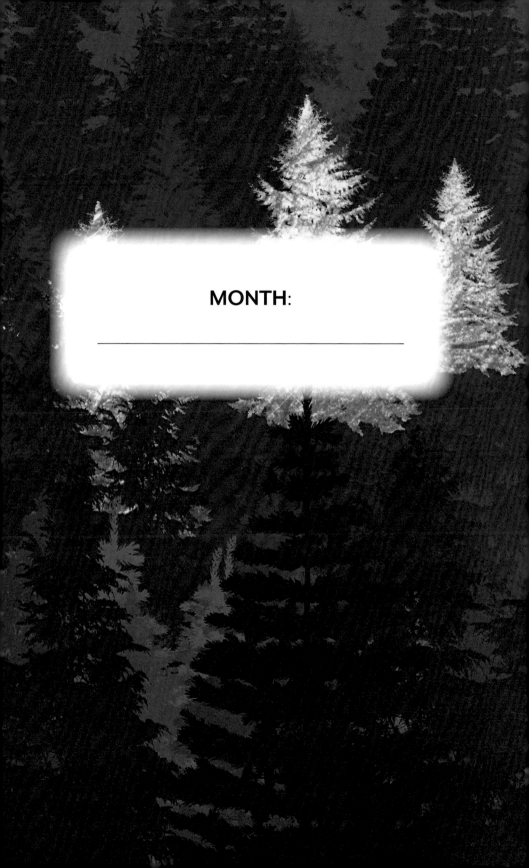

MONTH:

_____

WHAT IS the situation or circumstances that put you in the face of adversity, a traumatic time or difficult experience? This may include —but is not limited to— physical injury, illness, loss, financial issues, mental strain or emotional harm. What's your story?

_____

_____

_____

_____

_____

_____

_____

_____

_____

_____

_____

_____

_____

_____

_____

_____

_____

_____

_____

_____

_____

_____

_____

_____

_____

_____

_____

_____

USE THIS space to capture additional details about where you were, what you were doing and how this impacted your life. What other contributing factors or people were involved?

_____
_____
_____
_____
_____
_____
_____
_____
_____
_____
_____

WHAT WAS your mindset at the time? Use this area to jot down the feelings you processed. Did you feel fear, anger, frustration, overwhelm, devastation, disbelief or optimism? What feelings are coming up for you now about your story?

_____
_____
_____
_____
_____
_____
_____
_____
_____
_____
_____
_____
_____
_____
_____

WHAT DID you do next? Think back to that time and try to recall what you did next. What, if anything, would you do differently?

_____

_____

_____

_____

_____

_____

_____

_____

_____

_____

_____

_____

_____

WHAT WAS—or is—holding you back from moving forward on your path?

_____

_____

_____

_____

_____

_____

_____

_____

_____

_____

_____

_____

_____

_____

BREATHE

WHEN YOU find yourself stuck, stressed or emotionally heightened, you can try a technique called box breathing to gather and recenter yourself. It's a simple practice and easy to learn. It can help you increase your concentration, bring you back to the moment and feel grounded so you can continue moving forward on your path. You can do this anywhere at any time. Box breathing can be done lying down or seated.

FOUR BASIC STEPS FOR BOX BREATHING, EACH LASTING FOUR SECONDS:

1. Breathe in slowly for a count of four. Feel the air fill your lungs.

2. Hold your breath for a count of four, trying not to inhale or exhale.

3. Slowly release your breath, exhaling through your mouth for four seconds.

4. Hold your breath for another four-count.

Repeat these steps until you feel as though you've gathered yourself.

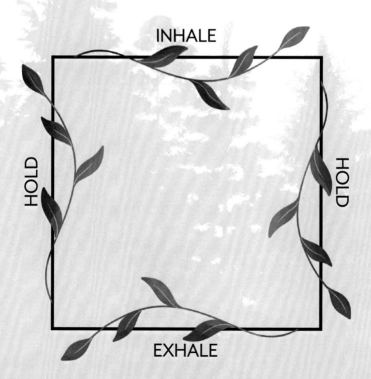

RESEARCH AND make a list of resources that can help you gain a better understanding of what information you'd like to gather. Ideas for your list could include books, personal development courses, workshops, retreats, conferences, websites, blogs, newsletters, mentorship, articles, videos, podcasts, apps and more. Be sure to connect with me on Instagram (@ginnypriem) where I'll share a variety of resources.

-
-
-
-
-
-
-
-
-

KEY LEARNINGS FROM RESOURCES:

_____

_____

_____

_____

_____

_____

_____

_____

_____

WHAT HAVE you discovered about yourself and your situation?

_____

_____

_____

_____

_____

_____

_____

_____

_____

WHAT ELSE would you like to gather and understand?

_____

_____

_____

_____

_____

_____

_____

_____

_____

WHAT'S NEXT on your path? Where would you like to go from here?

_____

_____

_____

_____

_____

_____

_____

_____

_____

_____

DO YOU engage in negative self-talk or hold a self-limiting belief you tell yourself or have told yourself in the past? If you're able, close your eyes and say this to yourself one time.

JOURNAL PROMPT: What did that bring up for you when you spoke to yourself in a negative way?

_____

_____

_____

_____

_____

_____

_____

_____

Take that negative self-talk and flip the script. Try saying the opposite. If that doesn't feel possible right now, try something 10% kinder. Close your eyes again and say this kinder thought to yourself three times, maybe even with a smile on your face.

JOURNAL PROMPT: How do you feel speaking in a more kind, positive way to yourself?

_____

_____

_____

_____

_____

_____

THINK ABOUT how your intentions or self-limiting thoughts have potentially been shaping your feelings and contributing to your overall happiness. What would you like to be intentional about that can bring you more peace and joy in your life?

_____

_____

_____

_____

_____

_____

_____

_____

_____

_____

_____

What you believe, you can become.
You're not defined by what happened to you,
but you can define your path forward.

WHAT DO you love about yourself or what are you learning to love?

_____

_____

_____

_____

_____

_____

_____

_____

_____

_____

WHEEL OF LIFE

THE WHEEL OF LIFE is a great tool to help you improve your life balance. It helps you quickly and graphically identify and gather information on the areas in your life to which you want to devote more energy, and helps you understand where you might want to intentionally cut back.

Start at the tip of the pie piece and color out to where you believe represents your current level of mastery in each of the areas.

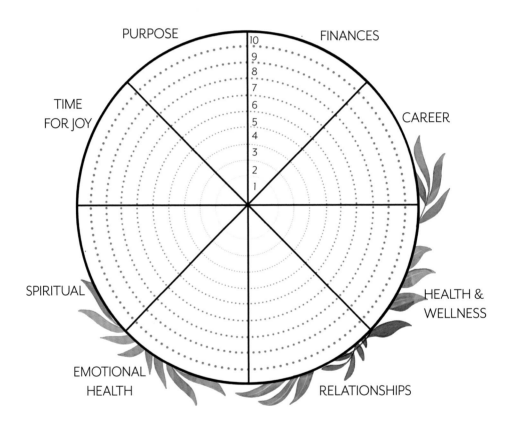

WHAT I'M proud of this month:

_____

_____

_____

_____

_____

INTENTIONS

INTENTION 1: _____
_____
_____
_____
_____

INTENTION 2: _____
_____
_____
_____
_____

INTENTION 3: _____
_____
_____
_____
_____

INTENTION 4: _____
_____
_____
_____
_____

INTENTION 5: _____
_____
_____
_____
_____

EMOTIONAL VIBRATION CHART

CONTEMPLATE THE emotions you've been feeling recently. On the chart, circle the emotions that most closely depict how you've felt over the past month or so.

ENLIGHTENMENT

PEACE

JOY

LOVE

REASON

ACCEPTANCE

WILLINGNESS

NEUTRALITY

COURAGE

PRIDE

ANGER

DESIRE

FEAR

GRIEF

APATHY

GUILT

SHAME

NOTES:

_____

_____

_____

_____

_____

_____

_____

_____

_____

_____

_____

_____

_____

_____

_____

_____

_____

_____

_____

_____

_____

NURTURE TRACKER

NURTURE

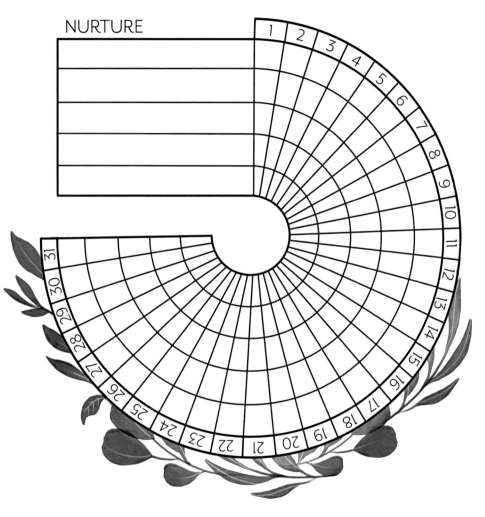

WHAT I'M proud of this month:

_____
_____
_____
_____
_____
_____
_____

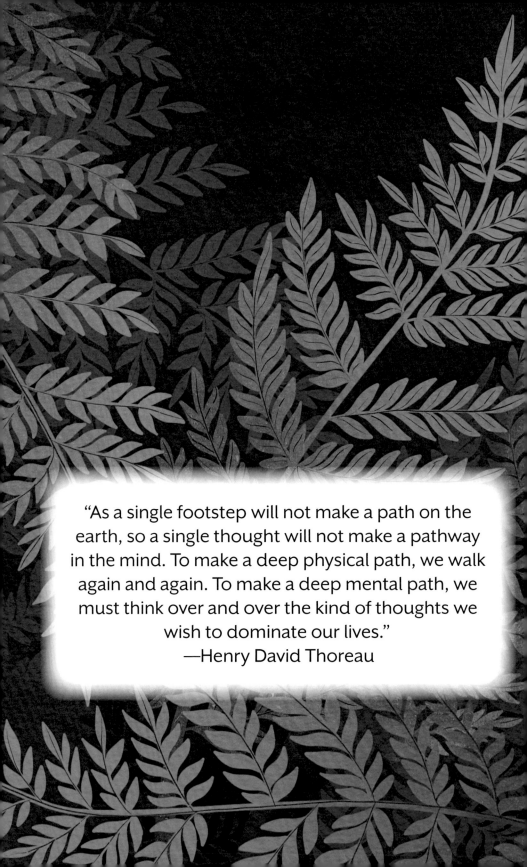

"As a single footstep will not make a path on the earth, so a single thought will not make a pathway in the mind. To make a deep physical path, we walk again and again. To make a deep mental path, we must think over and over the kind of thoughts we wish to dominate our lives."
—Henry David Thoreau

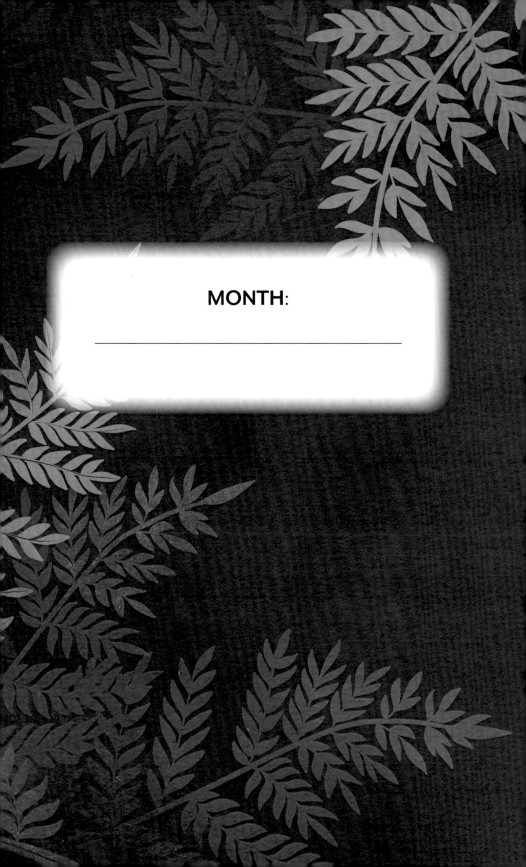

MONTH:

_____

WHAT IS the situation or circumstances that put you in the face of adversity, a traumatic time or difficult experience? This may include —but is not limited to— physical injury, illness, loss, financial issues, mental strain or emotional harm. What's your story?

_____

_____

_____

_____

_____

_____

_____

_____

_____

_____

_____

_____

_____

_____

_____

_____

_____

_____

_____

_____

_____

_____

_____

_____

_____

USE THIS space to capture additional details about where you were, what you were doing and how this impacted your life. What other contributing factors or people were involved?

_____

_____

_____

_____

_____

_____

_____

_____

_____

_____

_____

WHAT WAS your mindset at the time? Use this area to jot down the feelings you processed. Did you feel fear, anger, frustration, overwhelm, devastation, disbelief or optimism? What feelings are coming up for you now about your story?

_____

_____

_____

_____

_____

_____

_____

_____

_____

_____

_____

_____

_____

_____

WHAT DID you do next? Think back to that time and try to recall what you did next. What, if anything, would you do differently?

_____

_____

_____

_____

_____

_____

_____

_____

_____

_____

_____

_____

_____

WHAT WAS—or is—holding you back from moving forward on your path?

_____

_____

_____

_____

_____

_____

_____

_____

_____

_____

_____

_____

_____

BREATHE

WHEN YOU find yourself stuck, stressed or emotionally heightened, you can try a technique called box breathing to gather and recenter yourself. It's a simple practice and easy to learn. It can help you increase your concentration, bring you back to the moment and feel grounded so you can continue moving forward on your path. You can do this anywhere at any time. Box breathing can be done lying down or seated.

FOUR BASIC STEPS FOR BOX BREATHING, EACH LASTING FOUR SECONDS:

1. Breathe in slowly for a count of four. Feel the air fill your lungs.

2. Hold your breath for a count of four, trying not to inhale or exhale.

3. Slowly release your breath, exhaling through your mouth for four seconds.

4. Hold your breath for another four-count.

Repeat these steps until you feel as though you've gathered yourself.

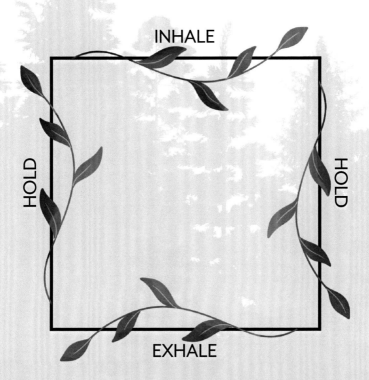

RESEARCH AND make a list of resources that can help you gain a better understanding of what information you'd like to gather. Ideas for your list could include books, personal development courses, workshops, retreats, conferences, websites, blogs, newsletters, mentorship, articles, videos, podcasts, apps and more. Be sure to connect with me on Instagram (@ginnypriem) where I'll share a variety of resources.

-
-
-
-
-
-
-
-
-
-

KEY LEARNINGS FROM RESOURCES:

_____

_____

_____

_____

_____

_____

_____

_____

_____

WHAT HAVE you discovered about yourself and your situation?

_____

_____

_____

_____

_____

_____

_____

_____

_____

WHAT ELSE would you like to gather and understand?

_____

_____

_____

_____

_____

_____

_____

_____

_____

WHAT'S NEXT on your path? Where would you like to go from here?

_____

_____

_____

_____

_____

_____

_____

_____

_____

DO YOU engage in negative self-talk or hold a self-limiting belief you tell yourself or have told yourself in the past? If you're able, close your eyes and say this to yourself one time.

JOURNAL PROMPT: What did that bring up for you when you spoke to yourself in a negative way?

_____

_____

_____

_____

_____

_____

_____

_____

Take that negative self-talk and flip the script. Try saying the opposite. If that doesn't feel possible right now, try something 10% kinder. Close your eyes again and say this kinder thought to yourself three times, maybe even with a smile on your face.

JOURNAL PROMPT: How do you feel speaking in a more kind, positive way to yourself?

_____

_____

_____

_____

_____

_____

_____

THINK ABOUT how your intentions or self-limiting thoughts have potentially been shaping your feelings and contributing to your overall happiness. What would you like to be intentional about that can bring you more peace and joy in your life?

_____
_____
_____
_____
_____
_____
_____
_____
_____
_____
_____

What you believe, you can become.
You're not defined by what happened to you,
but you can define your path forward.

WHAT DO you love about yourself or what are you learning to love?

_____
_____
_____
_____
_____
_____
_____
_____
_____
_____

WHEEL OF LIFE

THE WHEEL OF LIFE is a great tool to help you improve your life balance. It helps you quickly and graphically identify and gather information on the areas in your life to which you want to devote more energy, and helps you understand where you might want to intentionally cut back.

Start at the tip of the pie piece and color out to where you believe represents your current level of mastery in each of the areas.

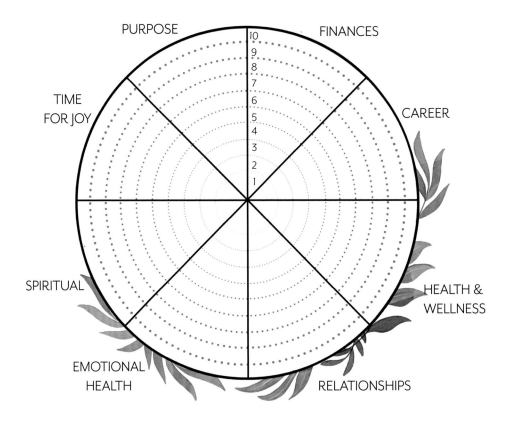

WHAT I'M proud of this month:

_____

_____

_____

_____

_____

INTENTIONS

INTENTION 1: _____
_____
_____
_____
_____

INTENTION 2: _____
_____
_____
_____
_____

INTENTION 3: _____
_____
_____
_____
_____

INTENTION 4: _____
_____
_____
_____
_____

INTENTION 5: _____
_____
_____
_____
_____

EMOTIONAL VIBRATION CHART

CONTEMPLATE THE emotions you've been feeling recently. On the chart, circle the emotions that most closely depict how you've felt over the past month or so.

ENLIGHTENMENT

PEACE

JOY

LOVE

REASON

ACCEPTANCE

WILLINGNESS

NEUTRALITY

COURAGE

PRIDE

ANGER

DESIRE

FEAR

GRIEF

APATHY

GUILT

SHAME

NOTES:

_____
_____
_____
_____
_____
_____
_____
_____
_____
_____
_____
_____
_____
_____
_____
_____
_____

NURTURE TRACKER

NURTURE

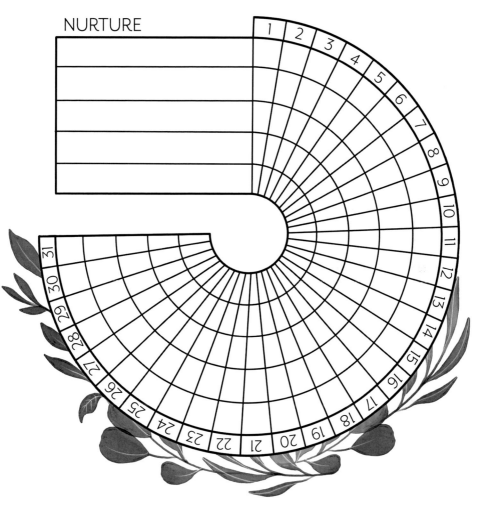

WHAT I'M proud of this month:

_____
_____
_____
_____
_____
_____
_____

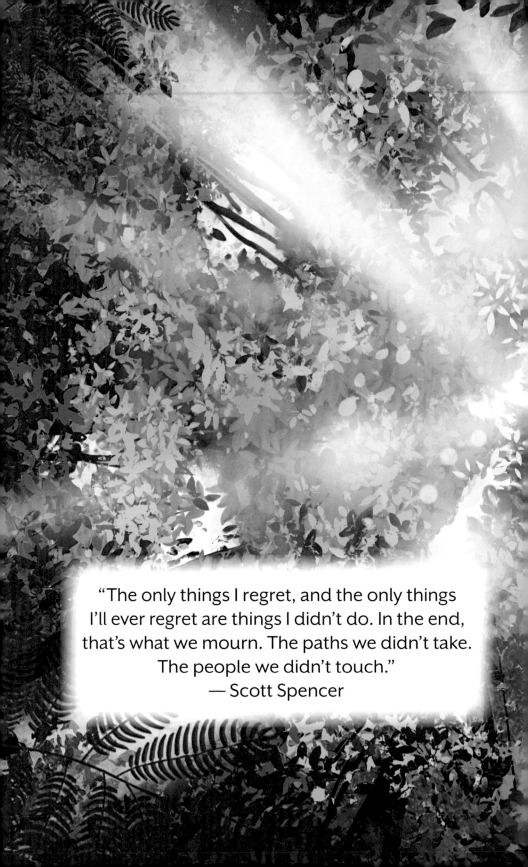

"The only things I regret, and the only things
I'll ever regret are things I didn't do. In the end,
that's what we mourn. The paths we didn't take.
The people we didn't touch."
— Scott Spencer

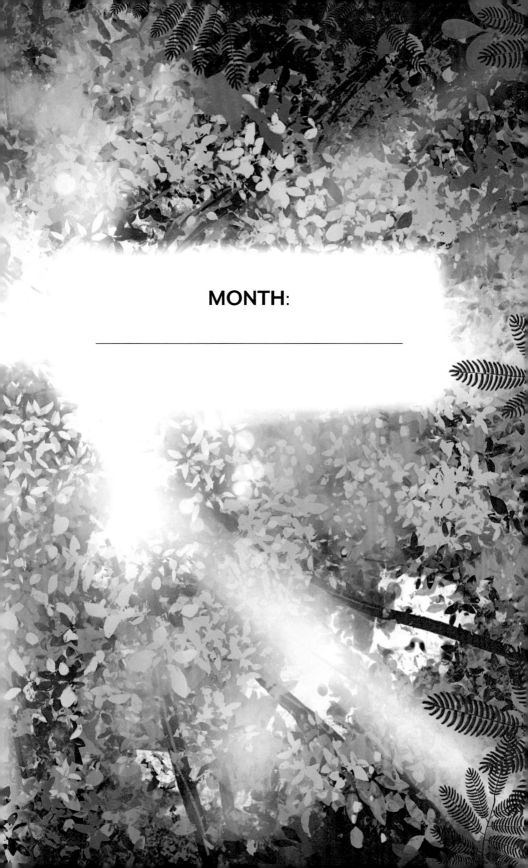

MONTH:

_____

WHAT IS the situation or circumstances that put you in the face of adversity, a traumatic time or difficult experience? This may include —but is not limited to— physical injury, illness, loss, financial issues, mental strain or emotional harm. What's your story?

_____

_____

_____

_____

_____

_____

_____

_____

_____

_____

_____

_____

_____

_____

_____

_____

_____

_____

_____

_____

_____

_____

_____

_____

_____

_____

_____

USE THIS space to capture additional details about where you were, what you were doing and how this impacted your life. What other contributing factors or people were involved?

_____
_____
_____
_____
_____
_____
_____
_____
_____
_____
_____

WHAT WAS your mindset at the time? Use this area to jot down the feelings you processed. Did you feel fear, anger, frustration, overwhelm, devastation, disbelief or optimism? What feelings are coming up for you now about your story?

_____
_____
_____
_____
_____
_____
_____
_____
_____
_____
_____
_____
_____

WHAT DID you do next? Think back to that time and try to recall what you did next. What, if anything, would you do differently?

_____
_____
_____
_____
_____
_____
_____
_____
_____
_____
_____
_____
_____
_____

WHAT WAS—or is—holding you back from moving forward on your path?

_____
_____
_____
_____
_____
_____
_____
_____
_____
_____
_____
_____
_____
_____
_____

BREATHE

WHEN YOU find yourself stuck, stressed or emotionally heightened, you can try a technique called box breathing to gather and recenter yourself. It's a simple practice and easy to learn. It can help you increase your concentration, bring you back to the moment and feel grounded so you can continue moving forward on your path. You can do this anywhere at any time. Box breathing can be done lying down or seated.

FOUR BASIC STEPS FOR BOX BREATHING, EACH LASTING FOUR SECONDS:

1. Breathe in slowly for a count of four. Feel the air fill your lungs.

2. Hold your breath for a count of four, trying not to inhale or exhale.

3. Slowly release your breath, exhaling through your mouth for four seconds.

4. Hold your breath for another four-count.

Repeat these steps until you feel as though you've gathered yourself.

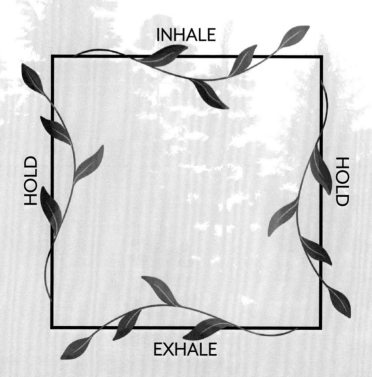

RESEARCH AND make a list of resources that can help you gain a better understanding of what information you'd like to gather. Ideas for your list could include books, personal development courses, workshops, retreats, conferences, websites, blogs, newsletters, mentorship, articles, videos, podcasts, apps and more. Be sure to connect with me on Instagram (@ginnypriem) where I'll share a variety of resources.

-
-
-
-
-
-
-
-
-

KEY LEARNINGS FROM RESOURCES:

_____
_____
_____
_____
_____
_____
_____
_____

WHAT HAVE you discovered about yourself and your situation?

_____
_____
_____
_____
_____
_____
_____
_____
_____
_____

WHAT ELSE would you like to gather and understand?

_____
_____
_____
_____
_____
_____
_____
_____

WHAT'S NEXT on your path? Where would you like to go from here?

_____
_____
_____
_____
_____
_____
_____
_____
_____
_____

DO YOU engage in negative self-talk or hold a self-limiting belief you tell yourself or have told yourself in the past? If you're able, close your eyes and say this to yourself one time.

JOURNAL PROMPT: What did that bring up for you when you spoke to yourself in a negative way?

_____
_____
_____
_____
_____
_____
_____
_____
_____

Take that negative self-talk and flip the script. Try saying the opposite. If that doesn't feel possible right now, try something 10% kinder. Close your eyes again and say this kinder thought to yourself three times, maybe even with a smile on your face.

JOURNAL PROMPT: How do you feel speaking in a more kind, positive way to yourself?

_____
_____
_____
_____
_____
_____
_____

THINK ABOUT how your intentions or self-limiting thoughts have potentially been shaping your feelings and contributing to your overall happiness. What would you like to be intentional about that can bring you more peace and joy in your life?

_____

_____

_____

_____

_____

_____

_____

_____

_____

_____

What you believe, you can become.
You're not defined by what happened to you,
but you can define your path forward.

WHAT DO you love about yourself or what are you learning to love?

_____

_____

_____

_____

_____

_____

_____

_____

_____

WHEEL OF LIFE

THE WHEEL OF LIFE is a great tool to help you improve your life balance. It helps you quickly and graphically identify and gather information on the areas in your life to which you want to devote more energy, and helps you understand where you might want to intentionally cut back.

Start at the tip of the pie piece and color out to where you believe represents your current level of mastery in each of the areas.

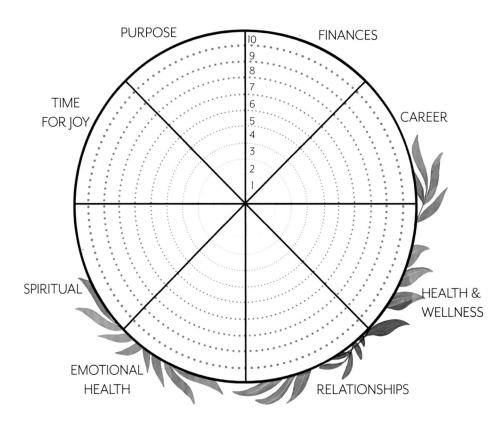

WHAT I'M proud of this month:

_____

_____

_____

_____

_____

INTENTIONS

INTENTION 1: _____
_____
_____
_____
_____

INTENTION 2: _____
_____
_____
_____
_____

INTENTION 3: _____
_____
_____
_____
_____

INTENTION 4: _____
_____
_____
_____
_____

INTENTION 5: _____
_____
_____
_____
_____

EMOTIONAL VIBRATION CHART

CONTEMPLATE THE emotions you've been feeling recently. On the chart, circle the emotions that most closely depict how you've felt over the past month or so.

ENLIGHTENMENT

PEACE

JOY

LOVE

REASON

ACCEPTANCE

WILLINGNESS

NEUTRALITY

COURAGE

PRIDE

ANGER

DESIRE

FEAR

GRIEF

APATHY

GUILT

SHAME

NOTES:

_____

_____

_____

_____

_____

_____

_____

_____

_____

_____

_____

_____

_____

_____

_____

_____

_____

_____

_____

_____

NURTURE TRACKER

NURTURE

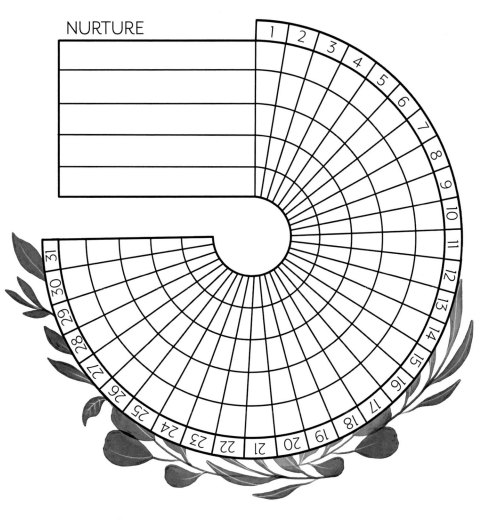

WHAT I'M proud of this month:

_____
_____
_____
_____
_____
_____
_____

NOTES

NOTES

NOTES

NOTES

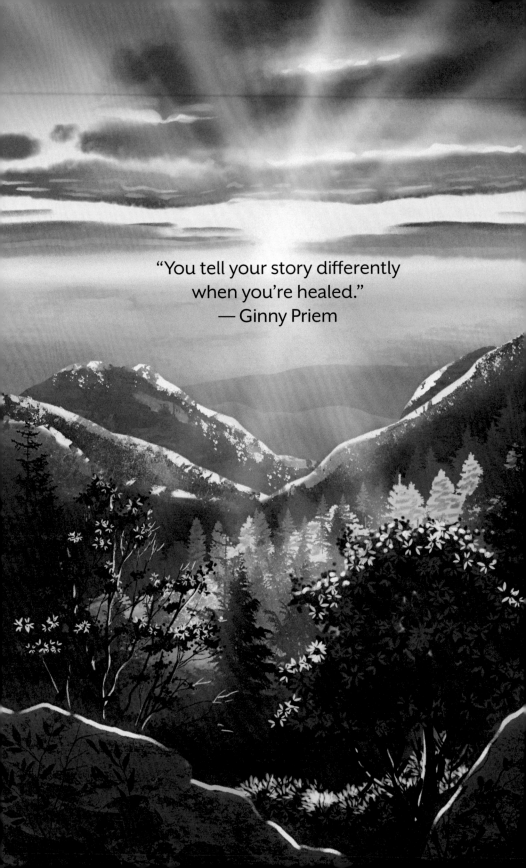

"You tell your story differently
when you're healed."
— Ginny Priem

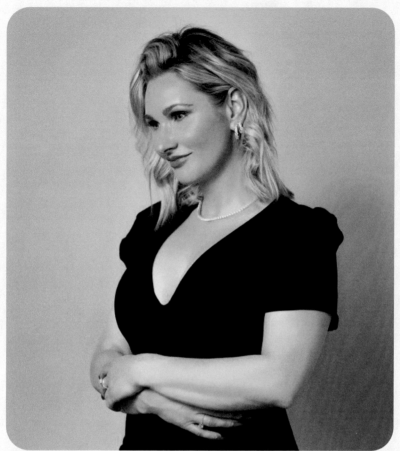
Photo by Profeshie

GINNY PRIEM has an extensive background including experience as a Master Certified Professional Life Coach and bestselling author. She is the host of the popular *Drinking With Gin* podcast and has over 15 years of speaking experience. In her #1 bestselling book, *You're My Favorite*, she shares the true story of her own personal traumatic end of a romantic relationship with a shocking twist: the man she thought was living in her house turned out to not be the man she thought he was at all. This jarring experience sent her on her own path of healing and growing. In discovering her own path forward, she created GINpath, which is the path that she developed, tested and implemented to help others in growing through adversity. She shares GINpath with her audiences on stage and in her latest book, *I'm My Favorite*. We all face tough times and have that one story, the one that we may not think is big enough to share or manage through, but it's what we do with these stories that really matters. *I'm My Favorite* is designed to help others grow forward on their own path. For more information about Ginny, visit her website at www.ginnypriem.com and connect with her on Instagram @ginnypriem.